Copyright © 2021 by James Kendall -All rights reserved.

No part of this book may be reproduced or transmitted in any form or by any means, electronic or mechanical, including photocopying and recording, or by any information storage and retrieval system, without permission in writing from the publisher. This is a work of fiction. Names, places, characters and incidents are either the product of the author's imagination or are used fictitiously, and any resemblance to any actual persons, living or dead, organizations, events or locales is entirely coincidental. The unauthorized reproduction or distribution of this copyrighted work is ilegal.

Please note the information contained within this document is for educational and entertainment purposes only. All effort has been executed to present accurate, up to date, reliable, complete information. No warranties of any kind are declared or implied. Readers acknowledge that the author is not engaged in the rendering of legal, financial, medical, or professional advice. The content within this book has been derived from various sources. Please consult a licensed professional before attempting any techniques outlined in this book. By reading this document, the reader agrees that under no circumstances is the author responsible for any losses, direct or indirect, that are incurred as a result of the use of the information contained within this document, including, but not limited to, errors, omissions, or inaccuracies.

CONTENTS

BREAKFAST RECIPES 6
    Grilled Ham Omelet 6
    Classic Bacon And Eggs Breakfast 6
    Quick Oat & Banana Pancakes 7
    Mexican Eggs On Haystacks 7
    Sausage And Mushroom Breakfast Skewers 8
    Chocolate Chip And Blueberry Pancakes 8
    Corn Cakes With Salsa And Cream Cheese 9

SNACK & DESSERT RECIPES 10
    Grilled Peaches 10
    Cinnamon Pancakes 10
    Fruity Skewers 11
    Blueberry Cream Cheese Pancakes 11
    Red Velvet Pancakes 12
    Pineapple 13
    Grilled Watermelon & Cream 13
    Chocolate-covered Grilled Strawberries 14
    Cinnamon Sugar Grilled Apricots 14
    Grilled Tomatoes With Garlic & Parmesan 15
    Grilled Pineapple With Coconut Sauce 15
    Shrimp & Pineapple Kabobs 16
    Banana Butter Kabobs 16
    Marshmallow Stuffed Banana 17
    Zucchini Rollups With Hummus 18
    Rum-soaked Pineapple 18
    Morning Waffles 19
    Grilled Fruit Kabobs 19
    Veggie Sliders 20
    Cinnamon Grilled Peaches 21
    Coconut-coated Pineapple 21
    Blueberry Waffles 22
    Almond Butter Pancakes 22
    Chocolate Waffles 23
    Nectarine 24
    Raspberry Pancakes 24
    Apple Crips In Foil 25
    Pumpkin Cream Cheese Pancakes 26
    Fruit Kabobs 26
    Apricots With Brioche 27
    Cheddar Cheese Pancakes 28
    Bacon-wrapped Peppers 28

APPETIZER & SIDE DISHES 29
Cauliflower Steaks 29
Zucchini Roulades 29
Charred Tofu 30
Parmesan Zucchini 31
Italian-seasoned Grilled Veggies 31
Sriracha Wings 32
Brussel Sprout Skewers 33
Garlicky Mushroom Skewers With Balsamic Vinegar 34
Grilled Brussels Sprouts 34
Grilled Zucchini 35
Grilled Mushroom Skewers 35
Grilled Butternut Squash 36
Lemony Green Beans 37
Grilled Veggies With Vinaigrette 37
Balsamic-glazed Carrots 38
Tarragon Asparagus 39
Veggie Burger 39
Cauliflower Zucchini Skewers 40
Butter Glazed Green Beans 41
Grilled Eggplant 41
Balsamic Bell Peppers 42

POULTRY RECIPES 43
Chicken Yakitori 43
Duck Veggie Kebobs 43
Glazed Chicken Drumsticks 44
Teriyaki Chicken Thighs 45
Seasoned Chicken Breast 45
Lemon And Rosemary Turkey And Zucchini Threads 46
Grilled Honey Chicken 47
Marinated Chicken Breasts 47
Lemon Grilled Chicken Thighs 48
Tequila Chicken 49
Chicken Burgers 49
Thyme Duck Breasts 50
Grilled Chicken Breast 51
Marinated Chicken Kabobs 51
Yucatan Chicken Skewers 52
Peach Glazed Chicken Breasts 53
Ketchup Glaze Chicken Thighs 54

FISH & SEAFOOD RECIPES 56
Lemony Salmon 56

Lemon-garlic Salmon 56
Soy Sauce Salmon 57
Blackened Salmon 58
Ginger Salmon 58
Herbed Salmon 59
Barbecue Squid 60
Salmon Lime Burgers 61
Grilled Scallops 62
Grilled Garlic Scallops 62
The Easiest Pesto Shrimp 63
Orange-glazed Salmon 63
Lemon Pepper Salmon With Cherry Tomatoes And Asparagus 64
Simple Mahi-mahi 64
Shrimp Skewers 65
Shrimp Kabobs 66

BEEF, PORK & LAMB RECIPES 67
    Spiced Lamb Chops 67
    Sweet Ham Kabobs 67
    Fajita Skewers 68
    Rosemary Lamb Chops 69
    Salisbury Steak 69
    Raspberry Pork Chops 70
    Greek Souzoukaklia 71
    Chimichurri Beef Skewers 71
    Spicy Pork Chops 72
    Garlicky Flank Steak 73
    Prosciutto-wrapped Pork Chops 74
    Glazed Pork Chops 75
    Garlicky Marinated Steak 75
    Grilled Pork Chops 76
    Filet Mignon 77
    Maple Pork Chops 77
    Beef Skewers 78
    Spiced Pork Tenderloin 79
    Pork Burnt Ends 80
    Hawaian Kebobs 81
    Lamb Steak 81
    Cheese Burgers 82
    Herbed Lemony Pork Skewers 83
    Grilled Lamb With Herbes De Provence 83
    Pork Kabobs 84
    Steak Skewers With Potatoes And Mushrooms 85

Grilled Lamb Chops 85
Chipotle Bbq Ribs 86
Margarita Beef Skewers 87
American Burger 87
Flank Steak 88
Lamb Kabobs 89
Honey Glazed Pork Chops 90
Lamb Skewers 90
Teriyaki Beef Skewers 91
Garlicy Lamb Chops 92

BREADS AND SANDWICHES 93
The Greatest Butter Burger Recipe 93
Simple Pork Chop Sandwich 93
Chicken Pesto Grilled Sandwich 94
Fish Tacos With Slaw And Mango Salsa 94
Buttery Pepperoni Grilled Cheese Sandwich 95
Cheesy Buffalo Avocado Sandwich 96

VEGETARIAN RECIPES 97
Garlicky Mixed Veggies 97
Grilled Tofu With Pineapple 97
Vinegar Veggies 98
Basil Pizza 99
Guacamole 99
Grilled Cauliflower 100

OTHER FAVORITE RECIPES 102
Mexican Scrambled Eggs 102
Lamb Burgers 102
Grilled Watermelon Salad With Cucumber And Cheese 103
Italian Panini 103
Grilled Zucchini And Feta Salad 104
Vegan Scrambled Eggs 105
Chocolate Panini 105
Spinach Scrambled Eggs 106
Sausage Scrambled Eggs 106

BREAKFAST RECIPES
Grilled Ham Omelet

Servings: 2
Cooking Time: 5 Minutes
Ingredients:
- 6 Eggs
- 2 Ham Slices, chopped
- 2 tbsp chopped Herbs by choice
- ¼ tsp Onion Powder
- 1 tbsp minced Red Pepper
- ¼ tsp Garlic Powder
- Salt and Pepper, to taste

Directions:
1. Preheat your grill to 350 degrees F.
2. In the meantime, whisk the eggs in a bowl and add the rest of the ingredients to it. Stir well to combine.
3. Open the grill and unlock the hinge.
4. Coat the griddle with some cooking spray and gently pour the egg mixture onto it.
5. With a silicone spatula, mix the omelet as you would in a skillet.
6. When it reaches your desired consistency, divide among two serving plates.
7. Enjoy!

Nutrition Info: Calories 271 ;Total Fats 17.5g ;Carbs 2.4g ;Protein 24g ;Fiber: 0.1g

Classic Bacon And Eggs Breakfast

Servings: 1
Cooking Time: 8 Minutes
Ingredients:
- 2 Eggs
- 2 Bacon Slices
- 2 Bread Slices
- Salt and Pepper, to taste

Directions:
1. Preheat your grill to 400 degrees F, and make sure that the kickstand is in position.
2. When the light goes on, add the bacon to the plate and lower the lid.
3. Let cook for 4 full minutes.
4. Open the lid and crack the eggs onto the plate. Season with salt and pepper.
5. Add the bread slices to the plate, as well.
6. Cook for 4 minutes, turning the bread and bacon (and the eggs if you desire) over ha-lfway through.
7. Transfer carefully to a plate. Enjoy!

Nutrition Info: Calories 434 ;Total Fats 19.6g ;Carbs 38.8g ;Protein 25.6g ;Fiber: 6g

Quick Oat & Banana Pancakes

Servings: 4
Cooking Time: 5 Minutes
Ingredients:
- ½ cup Oats
- ¼ cup chopped Nuts by choice (Walnuts and Hazelnuts work best)
- 1 large Ripe Banana, chopped finely
- 2 cups Pancake Mix

Directions:
1. Preheat your grill to medium and unlock the hinge. Open it flat on your counter.
2. Meanwhile, prepare the pancake mix according to the instruction on the package.
3. Stir in the remaining ingredients well.
4. Spray the griddle with some cooking spray.
5. Drop about ¼ cup onto the griddle.
6. Cook for a minute or two, just until the pancake begins to puff up.
7. Flip over and cook for another minute or so – the recipe makes about 16 pancakes.
8. Serve as desired and enjoy!

Nutrition Info: Calories 310 ;Total Fats 8g ;Carbs 56g ;Protein 14g ;Fiber: 8g

Mexican Eggs On Haystacks

Servings: 6
Cooking Time: 12 Minutes
Ingredients:
- ½ cup Breadcrumbs
- 3 ½ cups Store-Bought Hash Browns
- 2/3 cup Sour Cream
- 2 tsp Tex Mex Seasoning
- 6 Eggs
- 1/3 cup shredded Cheddar
- Salt and Pepper, to taste

Directions:
1. Preheat your grill to medium.
2. In the meantime, squeeze the hash browns to get rid of excess water, and place in a bowl.
3. Add the breadcrumbs, cheese, half of the Tex-Mex, and season with some salt and pepper.
4. Mix with your hands to combine.
5. Open the grill, unlock the hinge for the griddle, and lay it open. Spray with cooking spray.
6. Make six patties out of the hash brown mixture and arrange onto the griddle.

7. Cook for 7 minutes, flipping once, halfway through. Tarsnsfer to six serving plates.
8. Crack the eggs open onto the griddle, season with salt and pepper, and cook until they reach your preferred consistency.
9. Top the hash browns with the egg.
10. Combine the sourcream and remaining Tex Mex and top the eggs with it.
11. Enjoy!

Nutrition Info: Calories 340 ;Total Fats 21g ;Carbs 25g ;Protein 8.2g ;Fiber: 2g

Sausage And Mushroom Breakfast Skewers

Servings: 4
Cooking Time: 4 Minutes
Ingredients:
- 2 Italian Sausage Links
- 4 Whole White Button Mushrooms
- 1 Red Bell Pepper
- Salt and Pepper, to taste

Directions:
1. Soak four skewers in cold water for 2-3 minutes.
2. Preheat your grill to 375 degrees F.
3. Meanwhile, cut each sausage in eight pieces.
4. Quarter the mushrooms and cut the red pepper into eight pieces.
5. Sprinkle the mushrooms and pepper generously with salt and pepper.
6. Grab the skewers and thread the ingredients – sausage, mushroom, pepper, sausage, mushroom, sausage mushroom, pepper, sausage, mushroom, in that order.
7. Place onto the grill and lower the lid.
8. Cook for 4 minutes closed.
9. Serve alongside some bread and a favorite spread and enjoy.

Nutrition Info: Calories 118 ;Total Fats 9.1g ;Carbs 4g ;Protein 7.3g ;Fiber: 0.6g

Chocolate Chip And Blueberry Pancakes

Servings: 2
Cooking Time: 5 Minutes
Ingredients:
- 1 cup Pancake Mix
- ¼ cup Orange Juice
- 1/3 cup Fresh Blueberries
- ¼ cup Chocolate Chips
- ½ cup Water

Directions:
1. Preheat your grill to medium.

2. Meanwhile, combine the pancake mix with the orange juice and water.
3. Fold in the chocolate chips and blueberries.
4. Open the grill, unhinge, and lay the griddle onto your counter.
5. Spray with cooking spray.
6. Add about 1/6 of the batter at a time, to the griddle.
7. Cook until bubbles start forming on the surface, then flip over, and cook until the other side turns golden brown.
8. Serve and enjoy!

Nutrition Info: Calories 370 ;Total Fats 9g ;Carbs 66g ;Protein 3g ;Fiber: 3g

Corn Cakes With Salsa And Cream Cheese

Servings: 8
Cooking Time: 8 Minutes
Ingredients:
- ½ cup Cornmeal
- ¼ cup Butter, melted
- ½ cup Salsa
- 14 ounces canned Corn, drained
- 1 cup Milk
- 6 ounces Cream Cheese
- 1 ½ cups Flour
- 6 Eggs
- ¼ cup chopped Spring Onions
- 1 tsp Baking Powder
- Salt and Pepper, to taste

Directions:
1. In a bowl, whisk together the eggs, butter, cream cheese, and milk.
2. Whisk in the cornmeal, flour, baking powder, salt, and pepper.
3. Fold in the remaining ingredients and stir well to incorporate.
4. Preheat your grill to medium.
5. When the light is on, unlock the hinge and lower to your counter.
6. Spray the griddle with a nonstick spray.
7. Ladle the batter onto the griddle (about ¼ of cup per cake).
8. When the cakes start bubbling, flip them over and cook until golden brown.
9. Serve as desired and enjoy!

Nutrition Info: Calories 325 ;Total Fats 15g ;Carbs 35g ;Protein 11g ;Fiber: 3g

SNACK & DESSERT RECIPES

Grilled Peaches

Servings: 4
Cooking Time: 4 Minutes

Ingredients:
- 4 ripe peaches, halved and pitted
- 2 tablespoons maple syrup

Directions:
1. Place the water tray in the bottom of Power XL Smokeless Electric Grill.
2. Place about 2 cups of lukewarm water into the water tray.
3. Place the drip pan over water tray and then arrange the heating element.
4. Now, place the grilling pan over heating element.
5. Plugin the Power XL Smokeless Electric Grill and press the 'Power' button to turn it on.
6. Then press 'Fan" button.
7. Set the temperature settings according to manufacturer's directions.
8. Cover the grill with lid and let it preheat.
9. After preheating, remove the lid and grease the grilling pan.
10. Place the peach halves over the grilling pan, flesh side down.
11. Cover with the lid and cook for about 3-4 minutes.
12. Drizzle with maple syrup and serve.

Nutrition Info: (Per Serving):Calories 110 ;Total Fat 0.4 g ;Saturated Fat 0 g ;Cholesterol 0 mg ;Sodium 2 mg ;Total Carbs 27.2 g ;Fiber 2.3 g ;Sugar 25.7 g ;Protein 1.4 g

Cinnamon Pancakes

Servings: 2
Cooking Time: 4 Minutes

Ingredients:
- 1 large egg, beaten
- ¾ cup mozzarella cheese, shredded
- ½ tablespoon unsalted butter, melted
- 2 tablespoons all-purpose flour
- 2 tablespoons sugar
- ½ teaspoon ground cinnamon
- ½ teaspoon psyllium husk powder
- ¼ teaspoon baking powder
- ½ teaspoon vanilla extract
- For Topping:
- 1 teaspoon powdered sugar

- ¾ teaspoon ground cinnamon

Directions:
1. Turn the "Selector" knob to the "Griddle" side.
2. Preheat the bottom plate of the Cuisine GR Griddler at 350 degrees F.
3. In a medium bowl, put all ingredients and with a fork, mix until well combined.
4. Pour ¼ of the mixture into preheated Griddler and cook for about 2 minutes per side.
5. Cook more pancakes using the remaining batter.
6. Meanwhile, for topping: in a small bowl, mix together the sugar and cinnamon.
7. Place the pancakes onto serving plates and set aside to cool slightly.
8. Sprinkle with the cinnamon mixture and serve immediately.

Nutrition Info: (Per Serving): Calories 242 ;Total Fat 10.6 g ;Saturated Fat 4 g ;Cholesterol 106 mg ;Sodium 122 mg ;Total Carbs 24.1 g ;Fiber 2 g ;Sugar 0.3 g ;Protein 7.7 g

Fruity Skewers

Servings: 4
Cooking Time: 6 Minutes

Ingredients:
- 1 Pineapple, cut into chunks
- 12 Strawberries, halved
- 2 Mangos, cut into chunks
- ½ cup Orange Juice
- 2 tbsp Honey
- 1 tbsp Brown Sugar
- 1 tbsp Butter

Directions:
1. Preheat your grill to medium high.
2. Thread the fruit chunks onto soaked skewers.
3. Open the grill and place the skewers on the bottom grilling plate.
4. Cook for 3 minutes.
5. Flip over and cook for additional 3 minutes.
6. Meanwhile, combine the remaining ingredients in a small saucepan, and cook until slightly thickened.
7. Drizzle over the fruit skewers and serve. Enjoy!

Nutrition Info: Calories 180 ;Total Fats 4g ;Carbs 22g ;Protein 2g ;Fiber: 1g

Blueberry Cream Cheese Pancakes

Servings: 2
Cooking Time: 4 Minutes

Ingredients:
- 1 egg, beaten
- 1/3 cup Mozzarella cheese, shredded
- 1 teaspoon cream cheese, softened
- 1 teaspoon all-purpose flour
- ¼ teaspoon baking powder
- ¾ teaspoon powdered sugar
- ¼ teaspoon ground cinnamon
- ¼ teaspoon vanilla extract
- Pinch of salt
- 1 tablespoon fresh blueberries

Directions:
1. Turn the "Selector" knob to the "Griddle" side.
2. Preheat the bottom plate of the Cuisine GR Griddler at 350 degrees F.
3. In a bowl, place all ingredients except for blueberries and beat until well combined.
4. Fold in the blueberries.
5. Pour 1/2 of the mixture into preheated Griddler and cook for about 2 minutes per side.
6. Cook more pancakes using the remaining batter.
7. Serve warm.

Nutrition Info: (Per Serving): Calories 90 ;Total Fat 5 g ;Saturated Fat 2.7 g ;Cholesterol 97 mg ;Sodium 161 mg ;Total Carbs 25.7 g ;Fiber 2.8 g ;Sugar 1.2 g ;Protein 5.7 g

Red Velvet Pancakes

Servings: 2
Cooking Time: 4 Minutes

Ingredients:
- 2 tablespoons cacao powder
- 2 tablespoons Sugar
- 1 egg, beaten
- 2 drops super red food coloring
- ¼ teaspoon baking powder
- 1 tablespoon heavy whipping cream

Directions:
1. Turn the "Selector" knob to the "Griddle" side.
2. Preheat the bottom plate of the Cuisine GR Griddler at 350 degrees F.
3. In a medium bowl, put all ingredients and with a fork, mix until well combined.
4. Pour ½ of the mixture into preheated Griddler and cook for about 2 minutes per side.
5. Cook more pancakes using the remaining batter.
6. Serve warm.

Nutrition Info: (Per Serving): Calories 370 ;Total Fat 6 g ;Saturated Fat 3 g ;Cholesterol 92 mg ;Sodium 34 mg ;Total Carbs 33.2 g ;Fiber 1.5 g ;Sugar 0.2 g ;Protein 3.9 g

Pineapple

Servings: 6
Cooking Time: 10 Minutes
Ingredients:
- ¾ cup tequila
- ¾ cup brown sugar
- 1½ teaspoons vanilla extract
- ½ teaspoon ground cinnamon
- 1 large pineapple, peeled, cored and cut into 1-inch-thick slices

Directions:
1. Place tequila, sugar, vanilla and cinnamon in a bowl and mix well.
2. Place the water tray in the bottom of Power XL Smokeless Electric Grill.
3. Place about 2 cups of lukewarm water into the water tray.
4. Place the drip pan over water tray and then arrange the heating element.
5. Now, place the grilling pan over heating element.
6. Plugin the Power XL Smokeless Electric Grill and press the 'Power' button to turn it on.
7. Then press 'Fan" button.
8. Set the temperature settings according to manufacturer's directions.
9. Cover the grill with lid and let it preheat.
10. After preheating, remove the lid and grease the grilling pan.
11. Place the pineapple slices over the grilling pan.
12. Cover with the lid and cook for about 10 minutes, flipping and basting with tequila mixture occasionally.
13. Serve hot.

Nutrition Info: (Per Serving):Calories 225 ;Total Fat 0.2 g ;Saturated Fat 0 g ;Cholesterol 0 mg ;Sodium 8 mg ;Total Carbs 38.3 g ;Fiber 2.2 g ;Sugar 33 g ;Protein 0.8 g

Grilled Watermelon & Cream

Servings: 8
Cooking Time: 4 Minutes
Ingredients:
- 1 medium Watermelon
- 3 cups Whipped Cream
- 2 tbsp chopped Mint

Directions:

1. Preheat your grill to medium high.
2. Peel the melon and cut into wedges. Discard seeds if there are any.
3. Open the grill and arrange the wedges on top of the bottom plate.
4. Lower te lid and cook for 3-4 minutes.
5. Open and transfer to a cutting board.
6. Cut into smaller chunks and let cool.
7. Divide among 8 serving glasses.
8. Top with whipped cream and mint leaves.
9. Enjoy!

Nutrition Info: Calories 323 ;Total Fats 17.3g ;Carbs 44g ;Protein 4.4g ;Fiber: 2.2g

Chocolate-covered Grilled Strawberries

Servings: 4
Cooking Time: 6 Minutes
Ingredients:
- 12 Large Strawberries
- 3 ounces Chocolate
- 1 tbsp Butter

Directions:
1. Preheat your grill to 350 degrees F.
2. Clean and hull the strawberries.
3. When the green light appears, arrange the strawberries onto the plate.
4. Grill for about 6 minutes, rotating occasionally for even cooking.
5. Melt the chocolate and butter in a microwave. Stir to combine.
6. Coat the grilled strawberries with the melted chocolate and arrange on a platter.
7. Let harden before consuming.
8. Enjoy!

Nutrition Info: Calories 146 ;Total Fats 8g ;Carbs 18.3g ;Protein 1.4g ;Fiber: 1.6g

Cinnamon Sugar Grilled Apricots

Servings: 4
Cooking Time: 6 Minutes
Ingredients:
- 6 smallish Apricots
- 1 tbsp Butter, melted
- 3 tbsp Brown Sugar
- ½ tbsp Cinnamon

Directions:

1. Preheat your grill to 350 degrees F.
2. Cut the apricots in half and discard the seeds.
3. When ready, open the grill and coat with cooking spray.
4. Arrange the apricots and cook for 3 minutes.
5. Flip over and cook for 3 minutes more.
6. Meanwhile, whisk together the butter, sugar, and cinnamon.
7. Transfer the grilled apricots to a serving plate.
8. Drizzle the sauce over.
9. Enjoy!

Nutrition Info: Calories 92 ;Total Fats 2g ;Carbs 17g ;Protein 1g ;Fiber: 1g

Grilled Tomatoes With Garlic & Parmesan

Servings: 8
Cooking Time: 6 Minutes
Ingredients:
- ½ cup grated Parmesan Cheese
- 8 small Tomatoes, halved
- 1 tsp Garlic Powder
- 2 tbsp Olive Oil
- ¼ tsp Onion Powder
- Salt and Pepper, to taste

Directions:
1. Preheat your grill to 350 degrees F.
2. Combine the oil, garlic powder, onion powder, and salt and pepper, in a bowl.
3. Brush the tomatoes with this mixture.
4. Open the grill and arrange the tomatoes onto the plate.
5. Cook for 3 minutes, then flip over and cook for 2 more minutes.
6. Top with the parmesan cheese and cook for an additional minute.
7. Serve and enjoy!

Nutrition Info: Calories 78 ;Total Fats 5.6g ;Carbs 4.5g ;Protein 3.4g ;Fiber: 1g

Grilled Pineapple With Coconut Sauce

Servings: 4
Cooking Time: 8 Minutes
Ingredients:
- 1 large Pineapple
- 1 ½ tsp Cornstarch
- 2 tbsp Coconut Rum

- 1 tbsp Butter
- 1 tbsp Cream of Coconut

Directions:
1. Preheat your grill to medium high.
2. In the meantime, prepare the pineapple. Peel and slice into the size of your preference.
3. Thread the pineapple slices onto soaked skewers and open the grill.
4. Arrange on top of the bottom plate and grill for about 4 minutes per side.
5. In the meantime, whisk together the remaining ingredients in a saucepan.
6. Place over medium heat and cook until slightly thickened.
7. Serve the pineapple alongside the sauce.
8. Enjoy!

Nutrition Info: Calories 235 ;Total Fats 10g ;Carbs 34g ;Protein 2g ;Fiber: 3g

Shrimp & Pineapple Kabobs

Servings: 6
Cooking Time: 6 Minutes

Ingredients:
- 18 large Shrimp, cleaned
- 4 tbsp Honey
- 4 tbsp Soy Sauce
- 12 Pineapple Chunks
- 4 tbsp Balsamic Vinegar
- Salt and Pepper, to taste

Directions:
1. Thread the shrimp and pineapple onto skewers (no need to soak them) and place in a Ziploc bag.
2. In a bowl, whisk together the remaining ingredients.
3. Pour the mixture over the shrimp and pinapple.
4. Seal the bag and let marinate in the fridge for 15 minutes.
5. Meanwhile, preheat your grill to medium.
6. Once ready, open the grill and arrange the skewers onto the bottom plate.
7. Grill without lowering the lid, for 3 minutes per side.
8. Serve and enjoy!

Nutrition Info: Calories 61 ;Total Fats 1g ;Carbs 11g ;Protein 4g ;Fiber: 1g

Banana Butter Kabobs

Servings: 6
Cooking Time: 3 Minutes

Ingredients:
- 1 loaf (10 ¾ oz.) cake, cubed
- 2 large bananas, one-inch slices
- 1/4 cup butter, melted
- 2 tablespoons brown sugar
- 1/2 teaspoon vanilla extract
- 1/8 teaspoon ground cinnamon
- 4 cups butter pecan ice cream
- 1/2 cup butterscotch ice cream topping
- 1/2 cup pecans, chopped and toasted

Directions:
1. Thread the cake and bananas over the skewers alternately.
2. Whisk butter with cinnamon, vanilla, and brown sugar in a small bowl.
3. Brush this mixture over the skewers liberally.
4. Turn the "Selector" knob to the "Grill Panini" side.
5. Preheat the bottom grill of Cuisine Griddler at 300 degrees F and the upper grill plate on medium heat.
6. Once it is preheated, open the lid and place the banana skewers in the Griddler.
7. Close the griddler's lid and grill the skewers for 3 minutes.
8. Serve with ice cream, pecan, and butterscotch topping on top.

Nutrition Info: (Per Serving): Calories 419 ;Total Fat 19.7 g ;Saturated Fat 18.6 g ;Cholesterol 141 mg ;Sodium 193 mg ;Total Carbs 23.7 g ;Fiber 0.9 g ;Sugar 19.3 g ;Protein 5.2 g

Marshmallow Stuffed Banana

Servings: 1
Cooking Time: 8 Minutes

Ingredients:
- ¼ cup of chocolate chips
- 1 banana
- ¼ cup mini marshmallows

Directions:
1. Place a peeled banana over a 12 x 12-inch foil sheet.
2. Make a slit in the banana lengthwise and stuff this slit with chocolate chips and marshmallows.
3. Wrap the foil around the banana and seal it.
4. Turn the "Selector" knob to the "Griddle" side.
5. Prepare and preheat the bottom plate of Cuisine Griddler at 300 degrees F.
6. Once it is preheated, open the lid and place the banana in the Griddler.
7. Cook the banana in the Griddler for 4 minutes, flip and cook for another 4 minutes.

8. Unwrap and serve.

Nutrition Info: (Per Serving): Calories 372 ;Total Fat 11.8 g ;Saturated Fat 4.4 g ;Cholesterol 62 mg ;Sodium 871 mg ;Total Carbs 45.8 g ;Fiber 0.6 g ;Sugar 27.3 g ;Protein 4 g

Zucchini Rollups With Hummus

Servings: 4
Cooking Time: 3 Minutes
Ingredients:
- 2 medium Zucchini
- 6 tbsp Hummus
- 1 tbsp Olive Oil
- 1 Roasted Red Pepper, diced
- Salt and Pepper, to taste

Directions:
1. Preheat your grill to medium high.
2. Peel and slice the zucchini lengthwise.
3. Brush with olive oil and season with salt and pepper, generously.
4. Open the grill and arrange the zucchini slices on top.
5. Close the grill and cook for 2-3 minutes.
6. Transfer to a serving plate and let cool a bit until safe to handle.
7. Divide the hummus and red pepper among the grilled zucchini.
8. Roll up and secure the filling with a toothpick.
9. Serve and enjoy!

Nutrition Info: Calories 43 ;Total Fats 3.1g ;Carbs 3.6g ;Protein 1g ;Fiber: 1g

Rum-soaked Pineapple

Servings: 4
Cooking Time: 14 Minutes
Ingredients:
- 1/2 cup rum
- 1/2 cup packed brown sugar
- 1 teaspoon ground cinnamon
- 1 pineapple, cored and sliced
- Vanilla ice cream

Directions:
1. Mix run with cinnamon and brown sugar in a suitable bowl.
2. Pour this mixture over the pineapple rings and mix well.
3. Let them soak for 15 minutes and flip the pineapples after 7 minutes.

4. Turn the "Selector" knob to the "Grill Panini" side.
5. Preheat the bottom grill of Cuisine Griddler at 350 degrees F and the upper grill plate on medium heat.
6. Once it is preheated, open the lid and place the pineapple slices in the Griddler.
7. Close the griddler's lid and grill the pineapple for 5-7 minutes until lightly charred.
8. Serve with ice cream.

Nutrition Info: (Per Serving): Calories 427 ;Total Fat 31.1 g ;Saturated Fat 4.2 g ;Cholesterol 123 mg ;Sodium 86 mg ;Total Carbs 49 g ;Sugar 12.4 g ;Fiber 19.8 g ;Protein 13.5 g

Morning Waffles

Servings: 4
Cooking Time: 6 Minutes
Ingredients:
- ¼ cup all-purpose flour
- 2 tablespoons almond flour
- 1 teaspoon baking powder
- 2 tablespoons butter, melted
- 2 large eggs
- 2 ounces sour cream, softened
- ¼ cup powdered sugar
- 1½ teaspoons vanilla extract
- Pinch of salt

Directions:
1. Turn the "Selector" knob to the "Grill Panini" side.
2. Fix a waffle plates in the cuisine gr Griddler, preheat it at 350 degrees F and preheat the upper plate on medium heat.
3. In a bowl, add the butter and eggs and beat until creamy.
4. Add the cream, sugar, vanilla extract and salt and beat until well combined.
5. Add the flours and baking powder and beat until well combined.
6. Pour ¼ of the mixture into preheated Griddler, close the lid and cook for about 3 minutes.
7. Cook for waffle using the remaining batter.
8. Serve warm.

Nutrition Info: (Per Serving): Calories 217 ;Total Fat 18 g ;Saturated Fat 8.8 g ;Cholesterol 124 mg ;Sodium 173 mg ;Total Carbs 26.6 g ;Fiber 3.3 g ;Sugar 1.2 g ;Protein 5.3 g

Grilled Fruit Kabobs

Servings: 6
Cooking Time: 10 Minutes

Ingredients:
- 1 cup pineapple, cut into 1-inch pieces
- 1 banana, cut into 1-inch pieces
- 1 cup cantaloupe, cut into 1-inch pieces
- 1 cup fresh strawberries, hulled
- Coconut oil cooking spray
- 1 tablespoon maple syrup

Directions:
1. Thread the fruit pieces alternately onto pre-soaked wooden skewers.
2. Spray with cooking spray and then drizzle with maple syrup.
3. Place the water tray in the bottom of Power XL Smokeless Electric Grill.
4. Place about 2 cups of lukewarm water into the water tray.
5. Place the drip pan over water tray and then arrange the heating element.
6. Now, place the grilling pan over heating element.
7. Plugin the Power XL Smokeless Electric Grill and press the 'Power' button to turn it on.
8. Then press 'Fan" button.
9. Set the temperature settings according to manufacturer's directions.
10. Cover the grill with lid and let it preheat.
11. After preheating, remove the lid and grease the grilling pan.
12. Place the skewers over the grilling pan.
13. Cover with the lid and cook for about 10 minutes, flipping occasionally.
14. Serve immediately.

Nutrition Info: (Per Serving):Calories 56 ;Total Fat 0.2 g ;Saturated Fat 0 g ;Cholesterol 0 mg ;Sodium 5 mg ;Total Carbs 14.3 g ;Fiber 1.6 g ;Sugar 10.3 g ;Protein 0.7 g

Veggie Sliders

Servings: 10
Cooking Time: 7 Minutes

Ingredients:
- ½ Red Onion, diced
- ¾ cup cooked Quinoa
- 15 ounces canned Kidney
- ½ cup Walnuts, crushed or ground
- 1 shake Worcestershire Sauce
- 1 tbsp Chili Powder
- Salt and Pepper, to taste

Directions:
1. Preheat your grill to 350-375 degrees F.

2. Dump all of the ingredients in a bowl and mix well with your hands to incorporate the mixture.
3. Make about 10 small patties with your hands.
4. When ready, open the grill and coat with cooking spray.
5. Arrange the patties on top of the bottom plate.
6. Lower the lid and cook closed for about 6-7 minutes.
7. Serve on top of a lettuce leaf. Enjoy!

Nutrition Info: Calories 89 ;Total Fats 4.2g ;Carbs 9g ;Protein 4g ;Fiber: 3g

Cinnamon Grilled Peaches

Servings: 4
Cooking Time: 2 Minutes
Ingredients:
- 1/4 cup salted butter
- 1 tablespoon 1 teaspoon granulated sugar
- 1/4 teaspoon cinnamon
- 4 ripe peaches, pitted and sliced

Directions:
1. Mix sugar with butter and cinnamon in a bowl until smooth.
2. Turn the "Selector" knob to the "Grill Panini" side.
3. Preheat the bottom grill of Cuisine Griddler at 350 degrees F and the upper grill plate on medium heat.
4. Once it is preheated, open the lid and place the peach slices in the Griddler.
5. Close the griddler's lid and grill the peaches for 2 minutes.
6. Drizzle cinnamon butter on top and serve.

Nutrition Info: (Per Serving): Calories 401 ;Total Fat 8.9 g ;Saturated Fat 4.5 g ;Cholesterol 57 mg ;Sodium 340 mg ;Total Carbs 54.7 g ;Fiber 1.2 g ;Sugar 1.3 g ;Protein 5.3 g

Coconut-coated Pineapple

Servings: 6
Cooking Time: 6 Minutes
Ingredients:
- 1 Pineapple
- 2 tbsp Honey
- 1 tbsp Coconut Cream
- 1/3 cup Shredded Coconut

Directions:
1. Preheat your grill to medium high.

2. Meanwhile, peel and slice the coconut.
3. Thread each slice onto a soaked skewer.
4. Open the grill and arrange the skewers on top of the bottom plate.
5. Cook for 3 minutes per side.
6. Meanwhile, whisk together the honey and coconut cream.
7. Brush the pineapple with the mixture.
8. Place the coconut in a shallow bowl.
9. Coat the brushed pineapple with the coconut, on all sides.
10. Serve and enjoy!

Nutrition Info: Calories 75 ;Total Fats 20g ;Carbs 20g ;Protein 0g ;Fiber: 1g

Blueberry Waffles

Servings: 4
Cooking Time: 6 Minutes
Ingredients:
- ¼ cup all-purpose flour
- 1 teaspoon baking powder
- 2 tablespoons butter, melted
- 2 large eggs
- 2 ounces blueberry preserves
- ¼ cup powdered sugar
- 1½ teaspoons vanilla extract

Directions:
1. Turn the "Selector" knob to the "Grill Panini" side.
2. Fix a waffle plates in the cuisine gr Griddler, preheat it at 350 degrees F and preheat the upper plate on medium heat.
3. In a bowl, add the butter and eggs and beat until creamy.
4. Add the blueberry preserves, sugar, vanilla extract and salt and beat until well combined.
5. Add the flour and baking powder and beat until well combined.
6. Pour ¼ of the mixture into preheated Griddler, close the lid and cook for about 3 minutes.
7. Cook for waffle using the remaining batter.
8. Serve warm.

Nutrition Info: (Per Serving): Calories 215 ;Total Fat 8.5 g ;Saturated Fat 9.1 g ;Cholesterol 116 mg ;Sodium 131 mg ;Total Carbs 21.6 g ;Fiber 1.1 g ;Sugar 4.7 g ;Protein 3.8 g

Almond Butter Pancakes

Servings: 2
Cooking Time: 4 Minutes

Ingredients:
- 1 large egg, beaten
- 1/3 cup Mozzarella cheese, shredded
- 1 tablespoon sugar
- 2 tablespoons almond butter
- 1 teaspoon vanilla extract

Directions:
1. Turn the "Selector" knob to the "Griddle" side.
2. Preheat the bottom plate of the Cuisine GR Griddler at 350 degrees F.
3. In a medium bowl, put all ingredients and with a fork, mix until well combined.
4. Pour ¼ of the mixture into preheated Griddler and cook for about 2 minutes per side.
5. Cook for pancakes using the remaining batter.
6. Serve warm.

Nutrition Info: (Per Serving): Calories 253 ;Total Fat 12.3 g ;Saturated Fat 2 g ;Cholesterol 96 mg ;Sodium 65 mg ;Total Carbs 13.6 g ;Fiber 1.6 g ;Sugar 1.2 g ;Protein 7.9 g

Chocolate Waffles

Servings: 4
Cooking Time: 6 Minutes

Ingredients:
- ¼ cup all-purpose flour
- 2 tablespoons cocoa powder
- 1 teaspoon baking powder
- 2 tablespoons butter, melted
- 2 large eggs
- 2 ounces melted chocolate
- ¼ cup powdered sugar
- 1½ teaspoons vanilla extract

Directions:
1. Turn the "Selector" knob to the "Grill Panini" side.
2. Fix a waffle plates in the cuisine gr Griddler, preheat it at 350 degrees F and preheat the upper plate on medium heat.
3. In a bowl, add the butter and eggs and beat until creamy.
4. Add the cocoa powder, sugar, chocolate, vanilla extract and salt and beat until well combined.
5. Add the flours and baking powder and beat until well combined.
6. Pour ¼ of the mixture into preheated Griddler, close the lid and cook for about 3 minutes.
7. Cook for waffle using the remaining batter.
8. Serve warm.

Nutrition Info: (Per Serving): Calories 212 ;Total Fat 7.5 g ;Saturated Fat 9.1 g ;Cholesterol 216 mg ;Sodium 167 mg ;Total Carbs 24.1 g ;Fiber 0.2 g ;Sugar 2.1 g ;Protein 4 g

Nectarine

Servings: 2
Cooking Time: 6 Minutes
Ingredients:
- 2 medium nectarines, halved and pitted
- 1 tablespoon butter, melted
- 2 tablespoons honey
- ½ teaspoon ground nutmeg

Directions:
1. Brush the nectarine halves with butter evenly.
2. Place the water tray in the bottom of Power XL Smokeless Electric Grill.
3. Place about 2 cups of lukewarm water into the water tray.
4. Place the drip pan over water tray and then arrange the heating element.
5. Now, place the grilling pan over heating element.
6. Plugin the Power XL Smokeless Electric Grill and press the 'Power' button to turn it on.
7. Then press 'Fan" button.
8. Set the temperature settings according to manufacturer's directions.
9. Cover the grill with lid and let it preheat.
10. After preheating, remove the lid and grease the grilling pan.
11. Place the nectarine halves over the grilling pan.
12. Cook, uncovered for about 5-6 minutes, flipping and brushing with honey occasionally.
13. Transfer the nectarine halves onto a platter and set aside to cool.
14. Sprinkle with nutmeg and serve.

Nutrition Info: (Per Serving):Calories 180 ;Total Fat 6.4 g ;Saturated Fat 3.8 g ;Cholesterol 15 mg ;Sodium 42 mg ;Total Carbs 32.6 g ;Fiber 2.6 g ;Sugar 28.6 g ;Protein 1.7 g

Raspberry Pancakes

Servings: 2
Cooking Time: 4 Minutes
Ingredients:
- 1 egg, beaten
- 1 tablespoon cream cheese, softened
- ½ cup Mozzarella cheese, shredded
- 1 tablespoon powdered sugar
- ¼ teaspoon raspberry extract

- ¼ teaspoon vanilla extract

Directions:
1. Turn the "Selector" knob to the "Griddle" side.
2. Preheat the bottom plate of the Cuisine GR Griddler at 350 degrees F.
3. In a medium bowl, put all ingredients and with a fork, mix until well combined.
4. Pour ½ of the mixture into preheated Griddler and cook for about 2 minutes per side.
5. Cook more pancakes using the remaining batter.
6. Serve warm.

Nutrition Info: (Per Serving): Calories 269 ;Total Fat 5.2 g ;Saturated Fat 2.5 g ;Cholesterol 91 mg ;Sodium 88 mg ;Total Carbs 30.6 g ;Fiber 0 g ;Sugar 0.2 g ;Protein 5.2 g

Apple Crips In Foil

Servings: 8
Cooking Time: 20 Minutes
Ingredients:
- 4 Apples, sliced
- ½ cup Flour
- 4 tbsp Sugar
- 2 tsp Cinnamon
- ½ cup Quick Oats
- ½ cup Butter, melted
- ½ cup Brown Sugar
- ½ tsp Baking Powder

Directions:
1. Preheat your grill to 350 degrees F.
2. Prepare 4 aluminium foil squares (about 8x12 inches each).
3. Divide the apple slices among the foil and sprinkle with sugar and cinnamon.
4. In a bowl, combine the remaining ingredients well.
5. Divide the mixture evenly among the foil packets.
6. Carefully foil the packets, sealing so the filling stays inside.
7. When ready, open the grill and unlock the hinge.
8. Lay the griddle grate on top of your counter and place the foils there.
9. Cook for about 10 minutes.
10. Then, flip over, and cook for 10 minutes more.
11. Carefully open the packets and let sit for about 10 minutes before consuming.
12. Enjoy!

Nutrition Info: Calories 318 ;Total Fats 7g ;Carbs 51g ;Protein 2g ;Fiber: 3g

Pumpkin Cream Cheese Pancakes

Servings: 2
Cooking Time: 4 Minutes
Ingredients:
- 1 egg, beaten
- ½ cup Mozzarella cheese, shredded
- 1½ tablespoon sugar-free pumpkin puree
- 2 teaspoons heavy cream
- 1 teaspoon cream cheese, softened
- 1 tablespoon all-purpose flour
- 1 tablespoon Sugar
- ½ teaspoon pumpkin pie spice
- ½ teaspoon baking powder
- 1 teaspoon vanilla extract

Directions:
1. Turn the "Selector" knob to the "Griddle" side.
2. Preheat the bottom plate of the Cuisine GR Griddler at 350 degrees F.
3. In a medium bowl, put all ingredients and with a fork, mix until well **combined**.
4. Pour ½ of the mixture into preheated Griddler and cook for about 2 **minutes** per side.
5. Cook more pancakes using the remaining batter.
6. Serve warm.

Nutrition Info: (Per Serving): Calories 110 ;Total Fat 7.8 g ;Saturated Fat **3.1 g** ;Cholesterol 94 mg ;Sodium 82 mg ;Total Carbs 21.3 g ;Fiber 0.8g ;Sugar 1 g ;Protein 5.2 g

Fruit Kabobs

Servings: 6
Cooking Time: 9 Minutes
Ingredients:
- 1 tablespoon butter
- 1/2 cup apricot preserves
- 1 tablespoon water
- 1/8 teaspoon ground cinnamon
- 1/8 teaspoon ground nutmeg
- 3 nectarines, quartered
- 3 peaches, quartered
- 3 plums, quartered
- 1 loaf (10 ¾ oz.) lb. cake, cubed

Directions:

1. Take the first five ingredients in a small saucepan and stir cook for 3 minutes on medium heat.
2. Alternately thread the lb. cake and fruits on the skewers.
3. Brush these skewers with the apricot mixture.
4. Turn the "Selector" knob to the "Grill Panini" side.
5. Preheat the bottom grill of Cuisine Griddler at 350 degrees F and the upper grill plate on medium heat.
6. Once it is preheated, open the lid and place the fruit skewers in the Griddler.
7. Close the griddler's lid and grill the skewers for 4-6 minutes until lightly charred.
8. Serve.

Nutrition Info: (Per Serving): Calories 248 ;Total Fat 15.7 g ;Saturated Fat 2.7 g ;Cholesterol 75 mg ;Sodium 94 mg ;Total Carbs 38.4 g ;Fiber 0.3 g ;Sugar 10.1 g ;Protein 14.1 g

Apricots With Brioche

Servings: 4
Cooking Time: 5 Minutes

Ingredients:
- 8 ripe apricots
- 2 tablespoon butter
- 2 tablespoon sugar
- 4 brioche slices
- 2 tablespoon Honey
- 2 cup vanilla ice cream

Directions:
1. Toss the apricot halves with butter and sugar.
2. Turn the "Selector" knob to the "Grill Panini" side.
3. Preheat the bottom grill plate of Cuisine Griddler at 350 degrees F and the upper grill plate at medium heat.
4. Once it is preheated, open the lid and place the brioche slices in the Griddler.
5. Close the griddle's lid and grill the brioche for 3 minutes.
6. Transfer the grilled slices to a plate and keep them aside.
7. Now place the apricot slices in the Griddler, close the lid, and cook for 2 minutes.
8. Transfer the grilled apricots to the brioche slices and top with honey, sugar, and ice cream.
9. Serve.

Nutrition Info: (Per Serving): Calories 398 ;Total Fat 13.8 g ;Saturated Fat 5.1 g ;Cholesterol 200 mg ;Sodium 272 mg ;Total Carbs 53.6 g ;Fiber 1 g ;Sugar 1.3 g ;Protein 11.8 g

Cheddar Cheese Pancakes

Servings: 2
Cooking Time: 5 Minutes

Ingredients:
- 1 egg, beaten
- ½ cup Cheddar cheese, shredded
- Pinch of salt

Directions:
1. Turn the "Selector" knob to the "Griddle" side.
2. Preheat the bottom plate of the Cuisine GR Griddler at 350 degrees F.
3. Place about 1/8 cup of cheese in the bottom of the Griddler and top with half of the beaten egg.
4. Now, place 1/8 cup of cheese on top and cook for about 5 minutes.
5. Repeat with the remaining cheese and egg.
6. Serve warm.

Nutrition Info: (Per Serving): Calories 145 ;Total Fat 11.6 g ;Saturated Fat 6.6 g ;Cholesterol 112 mg ;Sodium 284 g ;Total Carbs 30.5 g ;Fiber 0 g ;Sugar 0.3 g ;Protein 9.8 g

Bacon-wrapped Peppers

Servings: 4
Cooking Time: 6 Minutes

Ingredients:
- 4 ounces Cream Cheese, softened
- 8 smallish Peppers
- 4 Bacon Slices

Directions:
1. Preheat your grill to 375 degrees F.
2. Cut of the top of the peppers and fiscard the seeds.
3. Fill the peppers with the cheese.
4. Cut the bacon slices in half, lengthwise, and wrap each pepper with it.
5. Open the grill and unlock the hinge.
6. Make sure the kickstand is in place.
7. Arrange the peppers onto the grill and cook for about 3 minutes.
8. Flip over and cook for another three minutes.
9. Serve and enjoy!

Nutrition Info: Calories 156 ;Total Fats 13g ;Carbs 5g ;Protein 1.1g ;Fiber: 6.2g

APPETIZER & SIDE DISHES
Cauliflower Steaks

Servings: 4
Cooking Time: 9 Minutes
Ingredients:
- 2 large heads cauliflower
- ¼ cup olive oil
- ½ teaspoons garlic powder
- ½ teaspoons paprika
- Kosher salt, to taste
- Black pepper, to taste
- 2 cups cheddar cheese, shredded
- Ranch dressing, for drizzling
- 8 cooked bacon slices, crumbled
- 2 tablespoons chives, chopped

Directions:
1. Mix olive oil, garlic powder, paprika, salt, and black pepper in a bowl
2. Slice the cauliflower into ¾ inch thick steaks and rub them with the olive oil mixture.
3. Turn the "Selector" knob to the "Grill Panini" side.
4. Preheat the bottom grill of Cuisine Griddler at 350 degrees F and the upper grill plate on medium heat.
5. Once it is preheated, open the lid and place the cauliflower steaks in the Griddler.
6. Close the griddler's lid and grill the steaks for 8 minutes until lightly charred.
7. Open the lid and drizzle bacon, cheddar cheese, ranch dressing and chives on top.
8. Cook for 1 minute until the cheese is melted.
9. Serve warm.

Nutrition Info: (Per Serving): Calories 278 ;Total Fat 3.8 g ;Saturated Fat 0.7 g ;Cholesterol 2 mg ;Sodium 620 mg ;Total Carbs 13.3 g ;Fiber 2.4 g ;Sugar 1.2 g ;Protein 5.4 g

Zucchini Roulades

Servings: 8
Cooking Time: 12 Minutes
Ingredients:
- 4 medium zucchinis
- 1 cup part-skim ricotta cheese
- ¼ cup Parmesan cheese, grated
- 2 tablespoons fresh basil, minced
- 1 tablespoon Greek olives, chopped

- 1 tablespoon capers, drained
- 1 teaspoon lemon zest, grated
- 1 tablespoon fresh lemon juice
- Salt and ground black pepper, as required

Directions:
1. Cut each zucchini into 1/8-inch thick slices lengthwise.
2. Place the water tray in the bottom of Power XL Smokeless Electric Grill.
3. Place about 2 cups of lukewarm water into the water tray.
4. Place the drip pan over water tray and then arrange the heating element.
5. Now, place the grilling pan over heating element.
6. Plugin the Power XL Smokeless Electric Grill and press the 'Power' button to turn it on.
7. Then press 'Fan" button.
8. Set the temperature settings according to manufacturer's directions.
9. After preheating, remove the lid and grease the grilling pan.
10. Place half of the zucchini slices over the grilling pan.
11. Cover with the lid and cook for about 2-3 minutes per side.
12. Transfer the zucchini slices onto a platter.
13. Repeat with the remaining slices.
14. Meanwhile, in a small bowl, place the remaining ingredients and mix well. Set aside.
15. Place about 1 tablespoon of cheese mixture on the end of each zucchini slice.
16. Roll up and secure each with a toothpick.
17. Serve immediately.

Nutrition Info: (Per Serving):Calories 70 ;Total Fat 3.4 g ;Saturated Fat 1.9 g ;Cholesterol 12 mg ;Sodium 131 mg ;Total Carbs 5.1 g ;Fiber 1.2 g ;Sugar 1.9 g ;Protein 5.8 g

Charred Tofu

Servings: 3
Cooking Time: 15 Minutes

Ingredients:
- 12 ounces extra-firm tofu, pressed, drained and cut into ½-inch thick slices
- Salt and ground black pepper, as required

Directions:
1. Season the tofu slices with salt and pepper.
2. Place the water tray in the bottom of Power XL Smokeless Electric Grill.
3. Place about 2 cups of lukewarm water into the water tray.
4. Place the drip pan over water tray and then arrange the heating element.
5. Now, place the grilling pan over heating element.
6. Plugin the Power XL Smokeless Electric Grill and press the 'Power' button to turn it on.
7. Then press 'Fan" button.

8. Set the temperature settings according to manufacturer's directions.
9. Cover the grill with lid and let it preheat.
10. After preheating, remove the lid and grease the grilling pan.
11. Place the mushrooms over the grilling pan.
12. Cover with the lid and cook for about 10-15 minutes, flipping once halfway through.
13. Serve warm.

Nutrition Info: (Per Serving):Calories 103 ;Total Fat 6.6 g ;Saturated Fat 0.6 g ;Cholesterol 0 mg ;Sodium 59 mg ;Total Carbs 2.3 g ;Fiber 0.5 g ;Sugar 0.6 g ;Protein 11.2 g

Parmesan Zucchini

Servings: 4
Cooking Time: 7 Minutes

Ingredients:
- 3 medium zucchinis, cut into ½-inch slices
- 2 tablespoons extra-virgin olive oil
- Salt and ground black pepper, as required
- ¼ cup parmesan cheese, shredded

Directions:
1. Brush the zucchini slices with oil and then sprinkle with salt and pepper.
2. Place the water tray in the bottom of Power XL Smokeless Electric Grill.
3. Place about 2 cups of lukewarm water into the water tray.
4. Place the drip pan over water tray and then arrange the heating element.
5. Now, place the grilling pan over heating element.
6. Plugin the Power XL Smokeless Electric Grill and press the 'Power' button to turn it on.
7. Then press 'Fan" button.
8. Set the temperature settings according to manufacturer's directions.
9. Cover the grill with lid and let it preheat.
10. After preheating, remove the lid and grease the grilling pan.
11. Place the zucchini slices over the grilling pan.
12. Cover with the lid and cook for about 5-7 minutes, flipping once halfway through.
13. Transfer the zucchini slices onto a plate and sprinkle with cheese.
14. Serve immediately.

Nutrition Info: (Per Serving):Calories 104 ;Total Fat 8.6 g ;Saturated Fat 1.9 g ;Cholesterol 4 mg ;Sodium 138 mg ;Total Carbs 5.1 g ;Fiber 1.6 g ;Sugar 2.5 g ;Protein 3.7 g

Italian-seasoned Grilled Veggies

Servings: 8
Cooking Time: 8 Minutes

Ingredients:
- 1 Zucchini, cut into chunks
- 1 Squash, cut into chunks
- 8 ounces Button Mushrooms, quartered
- 1 Red Bell Pepper, chopped
- 1 Red Onion, cut into chunks
- 2 tbsp Balsamic Vinegar
- 4 tbsp Olive Oil
- 2 tbsp Italian Seasoning
- 4 tbsp grated Parmesan Cheese
- Juice of 1 Lemon
- ½ tsp Garlic Powder

Directions:
1. Preheat your grill to medium-high heat.
2. In a bowl, place all of the ingredient, except the Parmesan Cheese.
3. With your hands, mix well so that each chunk of veggie is coated with oil and seasoning.
4. Thread the veggie chunks onto metal skewers (You can also use soaked wooden ones).
5. When the grill is ready, open the lid, and arrange the skewers onto the bottom plate.
6. Without covering the lid, cook for about 4 minutes.
7. Flip the skewers over and cook for another 3-4 minutes.
8. Serve sprinkled with Parmesan cheese and enjoy!

Nutrition Info: Calories 110 ;Total Fats 8g ;Carbs 7.5g ;Protein 3g ;Fiber: 2.5g

Sriracha Wings

Servings: 8
Cooking Time: 18 Minutes

Ingredients:
- For Wings:
- 3 pounds chicken wings
- 1 tablespoon canola oil
- 2 teaspoons ground coriander
- ½ teaspoon garlic salt
- ¼ teaspoon ground black pepper
- For Sauce:
- ½ cup fresh orange juice
- 1/3 cup Sriracha chili sauce
- ¼ cup butter, melted
- 3 tablespoons honey

- 2 tablespoons lime juice
- ¼ cup fresh cilantro, chopped

Directions:
1. For wings: in a bowl, place all ingredients and toss to coat well.
2. Cover the bowl and refrigerate for about 2 hours or overnight.
3. For sauce: in a bowl, place orange juice, chili sauce, butter, honey and lime juice and mix until well combined. Set aside.
4. Place the water tray in the bottom of Power XL Smokeless Electric Grill.
5. Place about 2 cups of lukewarm water into the water tray.
6. Place the drip pan over water tray and then, arrange the heating element.
7. Now, place the grilling pan over heating element.
8. Plugin the Power XL Smokeless Electric Grill and press the 'Power' button to turn it on.
9. Then press 'Fan" button.
10. Set the temperature settings according to manufacturer's directions.
11. Cover the grill with lid and let it preheat.
12. After preheating, remove the lid and grease the grilling pan.
13. Place the chicken wings over the grilling pan.
14. Cover with the lid and cook for about 15-18 minutes, flipping occasionally.
15. In the last 5 minutes of cooking, brush the wings with some of the sauce.
16. Transfer chicken into the bowl of the remaining sauce and toss to coat.
17. Garnish with cilantro and serve.

Nutrition Info: (Per Serving):Calories 432 ;Total Fat 20.1 g ;Saturated Fat 7.3 g ;Cholesterol 167 mg ;Sodium 258 mg ;Total Carbs 10.5 g ;Fiber 0.1 g ;Sugar 7.9 g ;Protein 49.5 g

Brussel Sprout Skewers

Servings: 8
Cooking Time: 7 Minutes
Ingredients:
- 24 Brussel Sprouts
- 2 tbsp Balsamic Glaze
- 4 tbsp Olive Oil
- ½ tsp Garlic Powder
- Salt and Pepper, to taste

Directions:
1. Preheat your grill to 375 degrees F.
2. In the meantime, trim the brussel sprouts and cut the in half.
3. Thread onto soaked wooden or metal skewers.
4. Drizzle with olive oil and sprinkle with the seasonings.
5. Place onto the bottom plate and cook uncovered for 4 minutes.

6. Turn over and cook for another 3 minutes or so.
7. Serve as desired and enjoy!

Nutrition Info: Calories 92 ;Total Fats 6g ;Carbs 6g ;Protein 1g ;Fiber: 2g

Garlicky Mushroom Skewers With Balsamic Vinegar

Servings: 4
Cooking Time: 4 Minutes

Ingredients:
- 2 pounds Button Mushrooms, halved
- 1 tbsp Tamari Sauce
- 2 tbsp Balsamic Vinegar
- ½ tsp Dried Thyme
- 2 large Garlic Cloves, minced
- Salt and Pepper, to taste

Directions:
1. Place the tamari, balsamic, thyme, and garlic, in a bowl.
2. Season with some salt and pepper and mix well to combine.
3. Add the mushrooms and toss to coat them well.
4. Cover the bowl and place in the fridge for about 30 minutes.
5. While the mushrooms are marinating, soak your wooden skewers in water to prevent burning.
6. Preheat your grill to 375 degrees F.
7. Thread the mushrooms onto your skewers and place on top of the bottom plate.
8. Grill for 2 minutes, then flip over, and grill for another two minutes, or until tender.
9. Serve and enjoy!

Nutrition Info: Calories 62 ;Total Fats 1g ;Carbs 9g ;Protein 7g ;Fiber: 2g

Grilled Brussels Sprouts

Servings: 2
Cooking Time: 9 Minutes

Ingredients:
- 1 lb. brussels sprouts, halved
- 3 tablespoons olive oil
- ¼ cup balsamic vinegar
- 1 tablespoon honey
- 1 tablespoon mustard
- 2 teaspoons crushed red pepper flakes
- Kosher salt

- ½ cup Parmesan, grated

Directions:
1. Mix oil, vinegar, honey, mustard, red pepper flakes, and salt in a bowl.
2. Toss in brussels sprout and toss well to coat.
3. Turn the "Selector" knob to the "Grill Panini" side.
4. Preheat the bottom grill of Cuisine Griddler at 350 degrees F and the upper grill plate on medium heat.
5. Once it is preheated, open the lid and place the brussels sprouts in the Griddler.
6. Close the griddler's lid and grill the brussels sprouts for 7-9 minutes until lightly charred.
7. Garnish with parmesan.

Nutrition Info: (Per Serving): Calories 121 ;Total Fat 3.8 g ;Saturated Fat 0.7 g ;Cholesterol 22 mg ;Sodium 620 mg ;Total Carbs 8.3 g ;Fiber 2.4 g ;Sugar 1.2 g ;Protein 5.4 g

Grilled Zucchini

Servings: 4
Cooking Time: 6 Minutes

Ingredients:
- 1-pound Zucchini
- 1 tbsp Lemon Juice
- 2 Garlic Cloves, minced
- 2 tbsp Olive Oil
- 1 tsp Italian Seasoning
- Salt and Pepper, to taste

Directions:
1. Trim and peel the zucchini. Cut into thick slices and place in a bowl.
2. Add all of the remaining ingredients and mix well so that the zucchini slices are completely coated.
3. Cover the bowl and place in the fridge for about one hour.
4. Menawhile, preheat your HB grill to 375 degrees F.
5. When the green light turns on, open the grill and place the zucchini slices onto the bottom plate.
6. Cook with the lid off, for three minutes. Flip over and cook for another three minutes.
7. Serve as desired and enjoy!

Nutrition Info: Calories 76 ;Total Fats 7g ;Carbs 1g ;Protein 0g ;Fiber: 0g

Grilled Mushroom Skewers

Servings: 6
Cooking Time: 3 Minutes

Ingredients:
- 2 pounds mushrooms, sliced
- 2 tablespoons balsamic vinegar
- 1 tablespoon soy sauce
- 3 garlic cloves, chopped
- 1/2 teaspoon thyme, chopped
- Salt and black pepper to taste

Directions:
1. Toss mushrooms with balsamic vinegar, soy sauce, garlic, thyme, black pepper and salt in a bowl.
2. Thread the mushroom slices on mini wooden skewers.
3. Turn the "Selector" knob to the "Grill Panini" side.
4. Preheat the bottom grill of Cuisine Griddler at 350 degrees F and the upper grill plate on medium heat.
5. Once it is preheated, open the lid and place mushroom skewers horizontally in the Griddler.
6. Close the griddler's lid and grill the mushrooms for 3 minutes.
7. Serve warm.

Nutrition Info: (Per Serving): Calories 418 ;Total Fat 15.7 g ;Saturated Fat 2.7 g ;Cholesterol 75 mg ;Sodium 94 mg ;Total Carbs 10.4 g ;Fiber 0.1 g ;Sugar 0.3 g ;Protein 4.9 g

Grilled Butternut Squash

Servings: 4
Cooking Time: 8 Minutes

Ingredients:
- 1 medium butternut squash, sliced
- 1 tablespoon olive oil
- 1 ½ teaspoons dried oregano
- 1 teaspoon dried thyme
- 1/2 teaspoon salt
- 1/4 teaspoon black pepper

Directions:
1. Peel and slice the squash into ½ inch thick slices.
2. Remove the center of the slices to discard the seeds.
3. Toss the squash slices with remaining ingredients in a bowl.
4. Turn the "Selector" knob to the "Grill Panini" side.
5. Preheat the bottom grill of Cuisine Griddler at 350 degrees F and the upper grill plate on medium heat.
6. Once it is preheated, open the lid and place the squash in the Griddler.
7. Close the griddler's lid and grill the squash for 8 minutes.

8. Serve warm.

Nutrition Info: (Per Serving): Calories 249 ;Total Fat 11.9 g ;Saturated Fat 1.7 g ;Cholesterol 78 mg ;Sodium 79 mg ;Total Carbs 41.8 g ;Fiber 1.1 g ;Sugar 20.3 g ;Protein 15 g

Lemony Green Beans

Servings: 3
Cooking Time: 6 Minutes
Ingredients:
- 2 tablespoons canola oil
- 2 garlic cloves, crushed
- 1 teaspoon red chili powder
- Salt, as required
- 1 pound fresh asparagus, trimmed

Directions:
1. In a bowl, place all ingredients except for lemon juice and toss to coat well.
2. Place the water tray in the bottom of Power XL Smokeless Electric Grill.
3. Place about 2 cups of lukewarm water into the water tray.
4. Place the drip pan over water tray and then arrange the heating element.
5. Now, place the grilling pan over heating element.
6. Plugin the Power XL Smokeless Electric Grill and press the 'Power' button to turn it on.
7. Then press 'Fan" button.
8. Set the temperature settings according to manufacturer's directions.
9. Cover the grill with lid and let it preheat.
10. After preheating, remove the lid and grease the grilling pan.
11. Place the asparagus over the grilling pan.
12. Cover with the lid and cook for about 5-6 minutes, turning occasionally.
13. Transfer the green beans into a bowl and drizzle with lemon juice.
14. Serve hot.

Nutrition Info: (Per Serving):Calories 118 ;Total Fat 9.7 g ;Saturated Fat 0.8 g ;Cholesterol 0mg ;Sodium 63 mg ;Total Carbs 7 g ;Fiber 3.5 g ;Sugar 2.9 g ;Protein 3.6 g

Grilled Veggies With Vinaigrette

Servings: 4
Cooking Time: 7 Minutes
Ingredients:
- Vinaigrette:
- 1/4 cup red wine vinegar
- 1 tablespoon Dijon mustard

- 1 tablespoon honey
- 1/2 teaspoon salt
- 1/8 teaspoon pepper
- 1/4 cup canola oil
- 1/4 cup olive oil
- Vegetables:
- 2 large sweet onions, sliced
- 2 yellow summer squash, sliced
- 2 large red peppers, seeded and sliced

Directions:
1. Whisk wine vinegar, Dijon mustard, honey, salt, black pepper olive oil and canola oil in a bowl.
2. Turn the "Selector" knob to the "Grill Panini" side.
3. Preheat the bottom grill of Cuisine Griddler at 350 degrees F and the upper grill plate on medium heat.
4. Once it is preheated, open the lid and place the vegetable slices in the Griddler.
5. Close the griddler's lid and grill the onions and peppers for 5 minutes and summer squash for 7 minutes.
6. Transfer the veggies to a serving plate and drizzle the vinaigrette on top.
7. Serve warm.

Nutrition Info: (Per Serving): Calories 341 ;Total Fat 4 g ;Saturated Fat 0.5 g ;Cholesterol 69 mg ;Sodium 547 mg ;Total Carbs 6.4 g ;Fiber 1.2 g ;Sugar 1 g ;Protein 10.3 g

Balsamic-glazed Carrots

Servings: 10
Cooking Time: 6 Minutes

Ingredients:
- 2 pounds Carrots, boiled for 3-4 minutes
- 3 tbsp Balsamic Vinegar
- 1 tsp ground Ginger
- 1 tsp Thyme
- 1 ½ tbsp Maple Syrup
- ½ tbsp Lime Juice
- Salt and Pepper, to taste

Directions:
1. Preheat your grill to 400 degrees F.
2. Meanwhile, cut the carrots in half lengthwise.
3. Place the remaining ingredients in a bowl and whisk well to combine.
4. Brush the carrots with the mixture, on all sides.

5. When the green light is on, open the grill and spray with some cooking spray.
6. Arrange the carrots on top of the bottom plate and cook for 3 minutes.
7. Flip over and cook for 3 more minutes on the other side.
8. Serve and enjoy!

Nutrition Info: Calories 50 ;Total Fats 1g ;Carbs 12g ;Protein 1g ;Fiber: 3g

Tarragon Asparagus

Servings: 4
Cooking Time: 4 Minutes
Ingredients:
- 2 lbs. fresh asparagus, trimmed
- 2 tablespoons olive oil
- 1 teaspoon salt
- 1/2 teaspoon black pepper
- 1/4 cup honey
- 4 tablespoons fresh tarragon, minced

Directions:
1. Liberally season the asparagus by tossing with oil, salt, pepper, honey, and tarragon.
2. Turn the "Selector" knob to the "Grill Panini" side.
3. Preheat the bottom grill of Cuisine Griddler at 300 degrees F and the upper grill plate on medium heat.
4. Once it is preheated, open the lid and place the asparagus in the Griddler.
5. Close the griddler's lid and grill the asparagus for 4 minutes.
6. Serve warm.

Nutrition Info: (Per Serving): Calories 148 ;Total Fat 15.7 g ;Saturated Fat 2.7 g ;Cholesterol 75 mg ;Sodium 94 mg ;Total Carbs 3.4 g ;Fiber 0.6 g ;Sugar 15 g ;Protein 14.1 g

Veggie Burger

Servings: 5
Cooking Time: 5 Minutes
Ingredients:
- 1 cup cooked brown rice
- 1 cup raw walnuts, finely chopped
- 1/2 tablespoons avocado oil
- 1/2 medium white onion, diced
- 1 tablespoon chili powder
- 1 tablespoon cumin powder
- 1 tablespoon smoked paprika

- 1/2 teaspoons sea salt
- 1/2 teaspoons black pepper
- 1 tablespoon coconut sugar
- 1 ½ cups cooked black beans, drained
- 1/3 cup panko bread crumbs
- 4 tablespoons BBQ sauce

Directions:
1. Add brown rice, walnuts, and all the veggies burger ingredients to a food processor.
2. Blend this mixture for 3 minutes then transfer to a bowl.
3. Make 5 patties out of this vegetable beans mixture.
4. Turn the "Selector" knob to the "Grill Panini" side.
5. Preheat the bottom grill of Cuisine Griddler at 350 degrees F and the upper grill plate on medium heat.
6. Once it is preheated, open the lid and place the veggie burgers in the Griddler.
7. Close the griddler's lid and grill the burgers for 5 minutes.
8. Serve warm.

Nutrition Info: (Per Serving): Calories 213 ;Total Fat 14 g ;Saturated Fat 8 g ;Cholesterol 81 mg ;Sodium 162 mg ;Total Carbs 23 g ;Fiber 0.7 g ;Sugar 19 g ;Protein 12 g

Cauliflower Zucchini Skewers

Servings: 8
Cooking Time: 10 Minutes

Ingredients:
- 4 large zucchinis sliced
- 1 head cauliflower, cut into florets
- Olive oil, for drizzling
- kosher salt, to taste
- Black pepper, to taste
- 1/4 cup crumbled feta

Directions:
1. Alternately, thread the cauliflower and zucchini slices on the wooden skewers.
2. Drizzle olive oil, black pepper and salt over the skewers.
3. Turn the "Selector" knob to the "Grill Panini" side.
4. Preheat the bottom grill of Cuisine Griddler at 300 degrees F and the upper grill plate on medium heat.
5. Once it is preheated, open the lid and place the skewers in the Griddler.
6. Close the griddler's lid and grill the cauliflower skewers for 10 minutes.
7. Garnish with feta cheese.
8. Serve.

Nutrition Info: (Per Serving): Calories 191 ;Total Fat 12.2 g ;Saturated Fat 2.4 g ;Cholesterol 110 mg ;Sodium 276 mg ;Total Carbs 5 g ;Fiber 0.9 g ;Sugar 1.4 g ;Protein 8.8 g

Butter Glazed Green Beans

Servings: 4
Cooking Time: 5 Minutes
Ingredients:
- 1-lb. fresh green beans, trimmed
- 1/2 teaspoon Cajun seasoning
- 1 tablespoon butter, melted

Directions:
1. Toss green beans with butter and Cajun seasoning in a bowl.
2. Turn the "Selector" knob to the "Grill Panini" side.
3. Preheat the bottom grill of Cuisine Griddler at 350 degrees F and the upper grill plate on medium heat.
4. Once it is preheated, open the lid and place the green beans in the Griddler.
5. Close the griddler's lid and grill the green beans for 5 minutes.
6. Serve warm.

Nutrition Info: (Per Serving): Calories 304 ;Total Fat 30.6 g ;Saturated Fat 13.1 g ;Cholesterol 131 mg ;Sodium 834 mg ;Total Carbs 21.4 g ;Fiber 0.2 g ;Sugar 0.3 g ;Protein 4.6 g

Grilled Eggplant

Servings: 4
Cooking Time: 8 Minutes
Ingredients:
- 2 small eggplants, half-inch slices
- 1/4 cup olive oil
- 2 tablespoons lime juice
- 3 teaspoons Cajun seasoning

Directions:
1. Liberally season the eggplant slices with oil, lemon juice, and Cajun seasoning.
2. Turn the "Selector" knob to the "Grill Panini" side.
3. Preheat the bottom grill of Cuisine Griddler at 300 degrees F and the upper grill plate on medium heat.
4. Once it is preheated, open the lid and place the eggplant slices in the Griddler.
5. Close the griddler's lid and grill the eggplant for 8 minutes until slightly charred.
6. Serve warm.

Nutrition Info: (Per Serving): Calories 172 ;Total Fat 11.1 g ;Saturated Fat 5.8 g ;Cholesterol 610 mg ;Sodium 749 mg ;Total Carbs 16.9 g ;Fiber 0.2 g ;Sugar 0.2 g ;Protein 3.5 g

Balsamic Bell Peppers

Servings: 4
Cooking Time: 10 Minutes
Ingredients:
- 1 pound small bell peppers, halved and seeded
- 1 tablespoon olive oil
- Salt and ground black pepper, as required
- 1 tablespoon balsamic vinegar

Directions:
1. Brush the bell pepper halves with oil and then sprinkle with salt and pepper.
2. Place the water tray in the bottom of Power XL Smokeless Electric Grill.
3. Place about 2 cups of lukewarm water into the water tray.
4. Place the drip pan over water tray and then arrange the heating element.
5. Now, place the grilling pan over heating element.
6. Plugin the Power XL Smokeless Electric Grill and press the 'Power' button to turn it on.
7. Then press 'Fan" button.
8. Set the temperature settings according to manufacturer's directions.
9. Cover the grill with lid and let it preheat.
10. After preheating, remove the lid and grease the grilling pan.
11. Place the bell pepper halves over the grilling pan.
12. Cover with the lid and cook for about 8-10 minutes, flipping once halfway through.
13. Transfer the bell pepper halves onto a plate and drizzle with vinegar.
14. Serve immediately.

Nutrition Info: (Per Serving):Calories 40 ;Total Fat 3.6 g ;Saturated Fat 0.5 g ;Cholesterol 0mg ;Sodium 40 mg ;Total Carbs 2.3 g ;Fiber 0.4 g ;Sugar 1.5 g ;Protein 0.3 g

POULTRY RECIPES
Chicken Yakitori

Servings: 4
Cooking Time: 6 Minutes
Ingredients:
- 2 tbsp Honey
- 1 tsp minced Garlic
- 1-pound boneless Chicken
- 1 tsp minced Ginger
- 4 tbsp Soy Sauce
- Salt and Pepper, to taste

Directions:
1. In a bowl, combine the honey, ginger, soy sauce, and garlic. Add some salt and pepper.
2. Cut the chicken into thick stripes and add them to the bowl.
3. Mix until the meat is completely coated with the marinade.
4. Cover the bowl and refrigerate for about one hour.
5. Preheat your grill to medium.
6. Thread the chicken onto metal (or soaked wooden) skewers and arrange onto the bottom plate.
7. Lower the lid and cook for about 6-7 minutes, depending on how well-cooked you prefer the meat to be.
8. Serve and enjoy!

Nutrition Info: Calories 182 ;Total Fats 9g ;Carbs 10g ;Protein 27g ;Fiber: 0.2g

Duck Veggie Kebobs

Servings: 2
Cooking Time: 7 Minutes
Ingredients:
- 8 ounces boneless and skinless Duck (breast is fine)
- 1/2 small Squash
- ½ Zucchini
- 1 small Red Bell Pepper
- ¼ Red Onion
- 2 tbsp Olive Oil
- 1 tbsp Balsamic Vinegar
- 2 tsp Dijon Mustard
- 2 tsp Honey
- Salt and Pepper, to taste

Directions:
1. Whisk together the oil, vinegar, mustard, honey, and some salt and pepper, in a bowl.
2. Cut the duck into chunks and dump into the bowl.
3. Mix to coat well and set aside. You can leave in the fridge for an hour or two, but if you are in a hurry, you can place on the grill straight away – it will taste great, as well.
4. Cut the veggies into chunks.
5. Plug the grill in, and set the temperature to 375 degrees F.
6. Thread the duck and veggies onto metallic skewers.
7. Open the grill and place on the bottom plate.
8. Lower the lid and cook for 5-8 minutes, depending on how done you want the meat to be.
9. Serve and enjoy!

Nutrition Info: Calories 250 ;Total Fats 10g ;Carbs 11g ;Protein 30g ;Fiber: 2g

Glazed Chicken Drumsticks

Servings: 12
Cooking Time: 25 Minutes

Ingredients:
- 1 (10-ounce) jar red jalapeño pepper jelly
- ¼ cup fresh lime juice
- 12 (6-ounce) chicken drumsticks
- Salt and ground black pepper, as required

Directions:
1. In a small saucepan, add jelly and lime juice over medium heat and cook for about 3-5 minutes or until melted.
2. Remove from the heat and set aside.
3. Sprinkle the chicken drumsticks with salt and black pepper.
4. Place the water tray in the bottom of Power XL Smokeless Electric Grill.
5. Place about 2 cups of lukewarm water into the water tray.
6. Place the drip pan over water tray and then arrange the heating element.
7. Now, place the grilling pan over heating element.
8. Plugin the Power XL Smokeless Electric Grill and press the 'Power' button to turn it on.
9. Then press 'Fan" button.
10. Set the temperature settings according to manufacturer's directions.
11. Cover the grill with lid and let it preheat.
12. After preheating, remove the lid and grease the grilling pan.
13. Place the chicken drumsticks over the grilling pan.
14. Cover with the lid and cook for about 15-20 minutes, flipping occasionally.
15. In the last 5 minutes of cooking, baste the chicken thighs with jelly mixture.
16. Serve hot.

Nutrition Info: (Per Serving):Calories 359 ;Total Fat 9.7 g ;Saturated Fat 2.6 g ;Cholesterol 150 mg ;Sodium 155 mg ;Total Carbs 17.1 g ;Fiber 0 g ;Sugar 11.4 g ;Protein 46.8 g

Teriyaki Chicken Thighs

Servings: 4
Cooking Time: 7 Minutes
Ingredients:
- 4 Chicken Thighs
- ½ cup Brown Sugar
- ½ cup Teriyaki Sauce
- 2 tbsp Rice Vinegar
- 1 thumb-sized piece of Ginger, minced
- ¼ cup Water
- 2 tsp minced Garlic
- 1 tbsp Cornstarch

Directions:
1. Place the sugar, teriyaki sauce, vinegar, ginger, water, and garlic, in a bowl.
2. Mix to combine well.
3. Transfer half of the mixture to a saucepan and set aside.
4. Add the chicken thighs to the bowl, and coat well.
5. Cover the bowl with wrap, and place in the fridge. Let sit for one hour.
6. Preheat your grill to medium.
7. In the meantime, place the saucepan over medium heat and add the cornstarch. Cook until thickened. Remove from heat and set aside.
8. Arrange the thighs onto the preheated bottom and close the lid.
9. Cook for 5 minutes, then open, brush the thickened sauce over, and cover again.
10. Cook for additional minute or two.
11. Serve and enjoy!

Nutrition Info: Calories 321 ;Total Fats 11g ;Carbs 28g ;Protein 31g ;Fiber: 1g

Seasoned Chicken Breast

Servings: 4
Cooking Time: 10 Minutes
Ingredients:
- 4 (4-ounce) boneless, skinless chicken breasts
- 1 teaspoon olive oil
- 1 teaspoon jerk seasoning

Directions:

1. Brush each chicken breast with olive oil and then rub with jerk seasoning.
2. Place the water tray in the bottom of Power XL Smokeless Electric Grill.
3. Place about 2 cups of lukewarm water into the water tray.
4. Place the drip pan over water tray and then arrange the heating element.
5. Now, place the grilling pan over heating element.
6. Plugin the Power XL Smokeless Electric Grill and press the 'Power' button to turn it on.
7. Then press 'Fan" button.
8. Set the temperature settings according to manufacturer's directions.
9. Cover the grill with lid and let it preheat.
10. After preheating, remove the lid and grease the grilling pan.
11. Place the chicken breasts over the grilling pan.
12. Cover with the lid and cook for about 3-5 minutes per side.
13. Serve hot.

Nutrition Info: (Per Serving):Calories 225 ;Total Fat 9.6 g ;Saturated Fat 2.5 g ;Cholesterol 101 mg ;Sodium 105 mg ;Total Carbs 0 g ; Fiber 0 g ;Sugar 0 g ;Protein 32.8 g

Lemon And Rosemary Turkey And Zucchini Threads

Servings: 4
Cooking Time: 7 Minutes

Ingredients:
- 1-pound Turkey Breasts, boneless and skinless
- 1 Large Zuchinni
- 2 tbsp Lemon Juice
- ½ tsp Lemon Zest
- ¼ cup Olive Oil
- 1 tbsp Honey
- 1 tbsp Fresh Rosemary
- ¼ tsp Garlic Powder
- Salt and Pepper, to taste

Directions:
1. Cut the Turkey into smaller chunks, and place inside a bowl.
2. Add the olive oil, lemon juice, zest, honey, rosemary, garlic powder, and some salt and pepper, to the bowl.
3. With your hands, mix well until the turkey is completely coated with the mixture.
4. Cover and let sit in the fridge for about an hour.
5. Wash the zucchini thoroughly and cut into small chunks. Season with salt and pepper.
6. Preheat your Grill to 350 – 375 degrees F.
7. Thread the turkey and zucchini onto soaked (or metal) skewers and arrange on the bottom plate.

8. Lower the lid and cook closed for 6-7 minutes.
9. Serve and enjoy!

Nutrition Info: Calories 280 ;Total Fats 23g ;Carbs 6g ;Protein 27g ;Fiber: 0.5g

Grilled Honey Chicken

Servings: 4
Cooking Time: 6 Minutes
Ingredients:
- Juice of 2 lemons
- ½ tablespoon Dijon mustard
- 1 tablespoon honey
- A dash of salt
- 2 whole chicken breasts

Directions:
1. Rub the chicken with honey, salt, Dijon and lemon juice.
2. Turn the "Selector" knob to the "Grill Panini" side.
3. Preheat the bottom grill of Cuisine Griddler at 350 degrees F and the upper grill plate on medium heat.
4. Once it is preheated, open the lid and place the chicken breasts in the Griddler.
5. Close the griddler's lid and grill the chicken for 6 minutes.
6. Serve warm.

Nutrition Info: (Per Serving): Calories 231 ;Total Fat 20.1 g ;Saturated Fat 2.4 g ;Cholesterol 110 mg ;Sodium 941 mg ;Total Carbs 30.1 g ;Fiber 0.9 g ;Sugar 1.4 g ;Protein 14.6 g

Marinated Chicken Breasts

Servings: 4
Cooking Time: 16 Minutes
Ingredients:
- ¼ cup extra-virgin olive oil
- 2 tablespoons fresh lemon juice
- 2 tablespoons maple syrup
- 1 garlic clove, minced
- Salt and ground black pepper, as required
- 4 (6-ounce) boneless, skinless chicken breasts

Directions:
1. For marinade: in a large bowl, add oil, lemon juice, maple syrup, garlic, salt and black pepper and beat until well combined.
2. In a large resealable plastic bag, place the chicken and marinade.

3. Seal the bag and shake to coat well.
4. Refrigerate overnight.
5. Place the water tray in the bottom of Power XL Smokeless Electric Grill.
6. Place about 2 cups of lukewarm water into the water tray.
7. Place the drip pan over water tray and then arrange the heating element.
8. Now, place the grilling pan over heating element.
9. Plugin the Power XL Smokeless Electric Grill and press the 'Power' button to turn it on.
10. Then press 'Fan" button.
11. Set the temperature settings according to manufacturer's directions.
12. Cover the grill with lid and let it preheat.
13. After preheating, remove the lid and grease the grilling pan.
14. Place the chicken breasts over the grilling pan.
15. Cover with the lid and cook for about 5-8 minutes per side.
16. Serve hot.

Nutrition Info: (Per Serving):Calories 460 ;Total Fat 25.3 g ;Saturated Fat 5.3 g ;Cholesterol 151 mg ;Sodium 188 mg ;Total Carbs 7.1 g ;Fiber 0.1 g ;Sugar 6.1 g ;Protein 49.3 g

Lemon Grilled Chicken Thighs

Servings: 4
Cooking Time: 6 Minutes
Ingredients:
- Juice and zest of 2 lemons
- 2 sprigs fresh rosemary, chopped
- 2 sprigs fresh sage, chopped
- 2 garlic cloves, smashed and chopped
- 1/4 teaspoon crushed red pepper
- 4 chicken thighs, trimmed
- Kosher salt, to taste

Directions:
1. Rub the chicken thighs with salt, oil, red pepper, garlic, sage, rosemary, lemon zest and juice.
2. Place the chicken in a bowl, cover and marinate for 1 hour for marination.
3. Turn the "Selector" knob to the "Grill Panini" side.
4. Preheat the bottom grill of Cuisine Griddler at 350 degrees F and the upper grill plate on medium heat.
5. Once it is preheated, open the lid and place 2 chicken thighs in the Griddler.
6. Close the griddler's lid and grill the chicken for 6 minutes.
7. Transfer them to a plate and grill the remaining thighs.
8. Serve warm.

Nutrition Info: (Per Serving): Calories 388 ;Total Fat 8 g ;Saturated Fat 1 g ;Cholesterol 153mg ;sodium 339 mg ;Total Carbs 8 g ;Fiber 1 g ;Sugar 2 g ;Protein 13 g

Tequila Chicken

Servings: 3
Cooking Time: 7 Minutes
Ingredients:
- 1/2 cup gold tequila
- 1 cup lime juice
- 1/2 cup orange juice
- 1 tablespoon chili powder
- 1 tablespoon minced jalapeno pepper
- 1 tablespoon minced fresh garlic
- 2 teaspoons kosher salt
- 1 teaspoon black pepper
- 3 boneless chicken breasts

Directions:
1. Mix tequila, lime juice, orange juice, chili powder, jalapeno pepper, garlic, black pepper and salt in a bowl.
2. Add chicken breasts to the tequila marinade, cover and marinate for 1 hour.
3. Turn the "Selector" knob to the "Grill Panini" side.
4. Preheat the bottom grill of Cuisine Griddler at 350 degrees F and the upper grill plate on medium heat.
5. Once it is preheated, open the lid and place the chicken breasts in the Griddler.
6. Close the griddler's lid and grill the chicken breasts for 7 minutes.
7. Serve warm.

Nutrition Info: (Per Serving): Calories 352 ;Total Fat 14 g ;Saturated Fat 2 g ;Cholesterol 65 mg ;Sodium 220 mg ;Total Carbs 15.8 g ;Fiber 0.2 g ;Sugar 1 g ;Protein 26 g

Chicken Burgers

Servings: 5
Cooking Time: 6 Minutes
Ingredients:
- 1 tablespoon butter, melted
- 1 small red onion, chopped
- 2 garlic cloves, chopped
- 2 tablespoons tomato paste
- 1 teaspoon sugar

- 1 tablespoon Worcestershire sauce
- 1 tablespoon hot sauce
- 1 1/4 pounds ground chicken
- 3 tablespoons olive oil
- 2 tablespoons honey

Directions:
1. Mix onion, butter, garlic, ground chicken, olive oil, honey, Worcestershire sauce, and sugar in a bowl.
2. Make the chicken patties out of this mixture.
3. Turn the "Selector" knob to the "Grill Panini" side.
4. Preheat the bottom grill of Cuisine Griddler at 350 degrees F and the upper grill plate on medium heat.
5. Once it is preheated, open the lid and place the patties in the Griddler.
6. Close the griddler's lid and grill the patties for 6 minutes.
7. Serve warm.

Nutrition Info: (Per Serving): Calories 529 ;Total Fat 17 g ;Saturated Fat 3 g ;Cholesterol 65 mg ;Sodium 391 mg ;Total Carbs 55 g ;Fiber 6 g ;Sugar 8 g ;Protein 41g

Thyme Duck Breasts

Servings: 2
Cooking Time: 16 Minutes
Ingredients:
- 2 shallots, sliced thinly
- 1 tablespoon fresh ginger, minced
- 2 tablespoons fresh thyme, chopped
- Salt and ground black pepper, as required
- 2 duck breasts

Directions:
1. In a large bowl, place the shallots, ginger, thyme, salt, and black pepper, and mix well.
2. Add the duck breasts and coat with marinade evenly.
3. Refrigerate to marinate for about 2-12 hours.
4. Place the water tray in the bottom of Power XL Smokeless Electric Grill.
5. Place about 2 cups of lukewarm water into the water tray.
6. Place the drip pan over water tray and then arrange the heating element.
7. Now, place the grilling pan over heating element.
8. Plugin the Power XL Smokeless Electric Grill and press the 'Power' button to turn it on.
9. Then press 'Fan" button.
10. Set the temperature settings according to manufacturer's directions.

11. Cover the grill with lid and let it preheat.
12. After preheating, remove the lid and grease the grilling pan, skin-side down.
13. Place the duck breast over the grilling pan.
14. Cover with the lid and cook for about 6-8 minutes per side.
15. Serve hot.

Nutrition Info: (Per Serving):Calories 337 ;Total Fat 10.1 g ;Saturated Fat 0 g ;Cholesterol 0 mg ;Sodium 80 mg ;Total Carbs 3.4 g ;Fiber 0 g ;Sugar 0.1 g ;Protein 55.5 g

Grilled Chicken Breast

Servings: 2
Cooking Time: 12 Minutes

Ingredients:
- 3 tablespoons olive oil
- 5 fresh basil leaves, torn
- 1 clove garlic, sliced
- 2 chicken breasts, boneless, skinless
- Kosher salt and black pepper, to taste

Directions:
1. Rub the chicken breasts with black pepper, salt, garlic, basil leaves and olive oil.
2. Turn the "Selector" knob to the "Grill Panini" side.
3. Preheat the bottom grill of Cuisine Griddler at 350 degrees F and the upper grill plate on medium heat.
4. Once it is preheated, open the lid and place the chicken breasts in the Griddler.
5. Close the griddler's lid and grill the skewers for 12 minutes.
6. Serve warm.

Nutrition Info: (Per Serving): Calories 453 ;Total Fat 2.4 g ;Saturated Fat 3 g ;Cholesterol 21 mg ;Sodium 216 mg ;Total Carbs 18 g ;Fiber 2.3 g ;Sugar 1.2 g ;Protein 23.2 g

Marinated Chicken Kabobs

Servings: 4
Cooking Time: 15 Minutes

Ingredients:
- 1/3 cup extra-virgin olive oil, divided
- 2 garlic cloves, minced
- 1 tablespoon fresh rosemary, minced
- 1 tablespoon fresh oregano, minced

- 1 teaspoon fresh lemon zest, grated
- ½ teaspoon red chili flakes, crushed
- 1 pound boneless, skinless chicken breast, cut into ¾-inch cubes
- 1¾ cups green seedless grapes, rinsed
- ½ teaspoon salt
- 1 tablespoon fresh lemon juice

Directions:
1. In small bowl, add ¼ cup of oil, garlic, fresh herbs, lemon zest and chili flakes and beat until well combined.
2. Thread the chicken cubes and grapes onto 12 metal skewers.
3. In a large baking dish, arrange the skewers.
4. Place the marinade and mix well.
5. Refrigerate to marinate for about 4-24 hours.
6. Place the water tray in the bottom of Power XL Smokeless Electric Grill.
7. Place about 2 cups of lukewarm water into the water tray.
8. Place the drip pan over water tray and then arrange the heating element.
9. Now, place the grilling pan over heating element.
10. Plugin the Power XL Smokeless Electric Grill and press the 'Power' button to turn it on.
11. Then press 'Fan" button.
12. Set the temperature settings according to manufacturer's directions.
13. Cover the grill with lid and let it preheat.
14. After preheating, remove the lid and grease the grilling pan.
15. Place the chicken skewers over the grilling pan.
16. Cover with the lid and cook for about 3-5 minutes per side or until chicken is done completely.
17. Remove from the grill and transfer the skewers onto a serving platter.
18. Drizzle with lemon juice and remaining oil and serve.

Nutrition Info: (Per Serving):Calories 310 ;Total Fat 20.1 g ;Saturated Fat 2.6 g ;Cholesterol 73 mg ;Sodium 351 mg ;Total Carbs 8.8 g ;Fiber 1.3 g ;Sugar 6.7 g ;Protein 24.6 g

Yucatan Chicken Skewers

Servings: 6
Cooking Time: 5 Minutes
Ingredients:
- 6 chicken thighs, boneless, cut in half lengthwise
- 1/2 cup orange juice
- 1/4 cup lime juice

- 2 tablespoons canola oil
- 2 tablespoons ancho chile powder
- 3 garlic cloves, chopped
- 2 tablespoons chipotle in adobo sauce, pureed
- Salt and black pepper, to taste

Directions:
1. Mix orange juice, lime juice, canola oil, chile powder, garlic, chipotle, black pepper and salt in a large bowl.
2. Add chicken thighs to the marinade then rub the chicken well.
3. Thread the chicken on the skewers and keep them aside.
4. Turn the "Selector" knob to the "Grill Panini" side.
5. Preheat the bottom grill of Cuisine Griddler at 350 degrees F and the upper grill plate on medium heat.
6. Once it is preheated, open the lid and place chicken skewers in the Griddler.
7. Close the griddler's lid and grill the chicken for 5 minutes.
8. Serve warm.

Nutrition Info: (Per Serving): Calories 284 ;Total Fat 25 g ;Saturated Fat 1 g ;Cholesterol 49 mg ;Sodium 460 mg ;Total Carbs 35 g ;Fiber 2 g ;Sugar 6 g ;Protein 26g

Peach Glazed Chicken Breasts

Servings: 4
Cooking Time: 10 Minutes

Ingredients:
- For Chicken:
- ¼ teaspoon ground cinnamon
- ¼ teaspoon ground nutmeg
- ¼ teaspoon ground cloves
- Salt, as required
- 4 (5-6-ounce) boneless skinless chicken breasts
- For Glaze:
- 1 peach, peeled and pitted
- 1 chipotle in adobo sauce
- 2 tablespoons fresh lemon juice

Directions:
1. In a bowl, place spices and salt and mix well.
2. Rub the chicken breasts with the spice mixture evenly.
3. For glaze: in a food processor, place peach, chipotle and lemon juice and pulse until pureed.

4. Transfer into a bowl and set aside.
5. Place the water tray in the bottom of Power XL Smokeless Electric Grill.
6. Place about 2 cups of lukewarm water into the water tray.
7. Place the drip pan over water tray and then arrange the heating element.
8. Now, place the grilling pan over heating element.
9. Plugin the Power XL Smokeless Electric Grill and press the 'Power' button to turn it on.
10. Then press 'Fan" button.
11. Set the temperature settings according to manufacturer's directions.
12. Cover the grill with lid and let it preheat.
13. After preheating, remove the lid and grease the grilling pan.
14. Place the chicken breasts over the grilling pan.
15. Cover with the lid and cook for about 8-10 minutes per side, brushing with the glaze after every 2 minutes.
16. Serve hot.

Nutrition Info: (Per Serving):Calories 287 ;Total Fat 10.7 g ;Saturated Fat 3 g ;Cholesterol 126 mg ;Sodium 163 mg ;Total Carbs 3.9 g ;Fiber 0.8 g ;Sugar 3.7 g ;Protein 41.5 g

Ketchup Glaze Chicken Thighs

Servings: 12
Cooking Time: 16 Minutes

Ingredients:

- ½ cup packed brown sugar
- 1/3 cup ketchup
- 1/3 cup low-sodium soy sauce
- 3 tablespoons sherry
- 1½ teaspoons fresh ginger root, minced
- 1½ teaspoons garlic, minced
- 12 (6-ounce) boneless, skinless chicken thighs

Directions:

1. In a small bowl, place all ingredients except for chicken thighs and mix well.
2. Transfer about 1 1/3 cups for marinade in another bowl and refrigerate.
3. In a zip lock bag, add the remaining marinade and chicken thighs.
4. Seal the bag and shake to coat well.
5. Refrigerate overnight.
6. Remove the chicken thighs from bag and discard the marinade.
7. Place the water tray in the bottom of Power XL Smokeless Electric Grill.
8. Place about 2 cups of lukewarm water into the water tray.

9. Place the drip pan over water tray and then arrange the heating element.
10. Now, place the grilling pan over heating element.
11. Plugin the Power XL Smokeless Electric Grill and press the 'Power' button to turn it on.
12. Then press 'Fan" button.
13. Set the temperature settings according to manufacturer's directions.
14. Cover the grill with lid and let it preheat.
15. After preheating, remove the lid and grease the grilling pan.
16. Place the chicken thighs over the grilling pan.
17. Cover with the lid and cook for about 6-8 minutes per side.
18. In the last 5 minutes of cooking, baste the chicken thighs with reserved marinade.
19. Serve hot.

Nutrition Info: (Per Serving):Calories 359 ;Total Fat 12.6 g ;Saturated Fat 3.6 g ;Cholesterol 151 mg ;Sodium 614 mg ;Total Carbs 8.3 g ;Fiber 0 g ;Sugar 7.6 g ;Protein 49.8 g

FISH & SEAFOOD RECIPES

Lemony Salmon

Servings: 4
Cooking Time: 14 Minutes

Ingredients:
- 2 garlic cloves, minced
- 1 tablespoon fresh lemon zest, grated
- 2 tablespoons butter, melted
- 2 tablespoons fresh lemon juice
- Salt and ground black pepper, as required
- 4 (6-ounce) boneless, skinless salmon fillets

Directions:
1. In a bowl, place all ingredients (except salmon fillets) and mix well.
2. Add the salmon fillets and coat with garlic mixture generously.
3. Place the water tray in the bottom of Power XL Smokeless Electric Grill.
4. Place about 2 cups of lukewarm water into the water tray.
5. Place the drip pan over water tray and then arrange the heating element.
6. Now, place the grilling pan over heating element.
7. Plugin the Power XL Smokeless Electric Grill and press the 'Power' button to turn it on.
8. Then press 'Fan" button.
9. Set the temperature settings according to manufacturer's directions.
10. Cover the grill with lid and let it preheat.
11. After preheating, remove the lid and grease the grilling pan.
12. Place the salmon fillets over the grilling pan.
13. Cover with the lid and cook for about 6-7 minutes per side.
14. Serve immediately.

Nutrition Info: (Per Serving):Calories 281 ;Total Fat 16.3 g ;Saturated Fat 5.2 g ;Cholesterol 90 mg ;Sodium 157 mg ;Total Carbs 1 g ;Fiber 0.2 g ;Sugar 0.3 g ;Protein 33.3 g

Lemon-garlic Salmon

Servings: 4
Cooking Time: 7 Minutes

Ingredients:
- 2 garlic cloves, minced
- 2 teaspoons lemon zest, grated
- 1/2 teaspoon salt
- 1/2 teaspoon fresh rosemary, minced
- 1/2 teaspoon black pepper

- 4 salmon fillets (6 oz.)

Directions:
1. Mix garlic with lemon zest, salt, rosemary and black pepper in a bowl
2. Leave this spice mixture for 15 minutes then rub it over the salmon with this mixture.
3. Turn the "Selector" knob to the "Grill Panini" side.
4. Preheat the bottom grill of Cuisine Griddler at 350 degrees F and the upper grill plate on medium heat.
5. Once it is preheated, open the lid and place the salmon in the Griddler.
6. Close the griddler's lid and grill the salmon for 7 minutes.
7. Serve warm.

Nutrition Info: (Per Serving): Calories 246 ;Total Fat 7.4 g ;Saturated Fat 4.6 g ;Cholesterol 105 mg ;Sodium 353 mg ;Total Carbs 19.4 g ;Sugar 6.5 g ;Fiber 2.7 g ;Protein 37.2 g

Soy Sauce Salmon

Servings: 4

Cooking Time: 10 Minutes

Ingredients:
- 2 tablespoons scallions, chopped
- ¾ teaspoon fresh ginger, minced
- 1 garlic clove, minced
- ½ teaspoon dried dill weed, crushed
- ¼ cup olive oil
- 2 tablespoons balsamic vinegar
- 2 tablespoons low-sodium soy sauce
- 4 (5-ounce) boneless salmon fillets

Directions:
1. Add all ingredients except for salmon in a large bowl and mix well.
2. Add salmon and coat with marinade generously.
3. Cover and refrigerate to marinate for at least 4-5 hours.
4. Place the water tray in the bottom of Power XL Smokeless Electric Grill.
5. Place about 2 cups of lukewarm water into the water tray.
6. Place the drip pan over water tray and then arrange the heating element.
7. Now, place the grilling pan over heating element.
8. Plugin the Power XL Smokeless Electric Grill and press the 'Power' button to turn it on.
9. Then press 'Fan' button.
10. Set the temperature settings according to manufacturer's directions.
11. Cover the grill with lid and let it preheat.
12. After preheating, remove the lid and grease the grilling pan.
13. Place the salmon fillets over the grilling pan.

14. Cover with the lid and cook for about 5 minutes per side.
15. Serve hot.

Nutrition Info: (Per Serving):Calories 303 ;Total Fat 21.4 g ;Saturated Fat 3.1 g ;Cholesterol 63 mg ;Sodium 504 mg ;Total Carbs 1.4 g ;Fiber 0.2 g ;Sugar 0.6 g ;Protein 28.2 g

Blackened Salmon

Servings: 2
Cooking Time: 6 Minutes
Ingredients:
- 1 lb. salmon fillets
- 3 tablespoons butter, melted
- 1 tablespoon lemon pepper
- 1 teaspoon seasoned salt
- 1½ tablespoon smoked paprika
- 1 teaspoon cayenne pepper
- ¾ teaspoon onion salt
- ½ teaspoon dry basil
- ½ teaspoon ground white pepper
- ½ teaspoon ground black pepper
- ¼ teaspoon dry oregano
- ¼ teaspoon ancho chili powder

Directions:
1. Liberally season the salmon fillets with butter and other ingredients.
2. Turn the "Selector" knob to the "Grill Panini" side.
3. Preheat the bottom grill of Cuisine Griddler at 350 degrees F and the upper grill plate on medium heat.
4. Once it is preheated, open the lid and place the salmon fillets in the Griddler.
5. Close the griddler's lid and grill the fish fillets for 6 minutes.
6. Serve warm.

Nutrition Info: (Per Serving): Calories 378 ;Total Fat 7 g ;Saturated Fat 8.1 g ;Cholesterol 230 mg ;Sodium 316 mg ;Total Carbs 16.2 g ;Sugar 0.2 g ;Fiber 0.3 g ;Protein 26 g

Ginger Salmon

Servings: 3
Cooking Time: 8 Minutes
Ingredients:
- Sauce:
- ¼ tablespoons rice vinegar

- 1 teaspoons sugar
- 1/8 teaspoon salt
- ¼ tablespoon lime zest, grated
- 1/8 cup lime juice
- ½ tablespoon olive oil
- 1/8 teaspoon ground coriander
- 1/8 teaspoon ground black pepper
- 1/8 cup cilantro, chopped
- ¼ tablespoon onion, chopped
- ½ teaspoon ginger root, minced
- 1 garlic clove, minced
- 1 small cucumber, peeled, chopped
- Salmon:
- 2 tablespoons gingerroot, minced
- ¼ tablespoon lime juice
- ¼ tablespoon olive oil
- Salt, to taste
- Black pepper, to taste
- 3 (6 oz.) salmon fillets

Directions:
1. Start by blending the cucumber with all the sauce ingredients in a blender until smooth.
2. Season and rub the salmon fillets with ginger, oil, salt, black pepper, lime juice.
3. Turn the "Selector" knob to the "Grill Panini" side.
4. Preheat the bottom grill of Cuisine Griddler at 350 degrees F and the upper grill plate on medium heat.
5. Once it is preheated, open the lid and place the salmon fillets in the Griddler.
6. Close the griddler's lid and grill the salmon fillets for 8 minutes.
7. Serve warm with cucumber sauce.

Nutrition Info: (Per Serving): Calories 457 ;Total Fat 19.1 g ;Saturated Fat 11 g ;Cholesterol 262 mg ;Sodium 557 mg ;Total Carbs 18.9 g ;Sugar 1.2 g ;Fiber 1.7 g ;Protein 32.5 g

Herbed Salmon

Servings: 4
Cooking Time: 8 Minutes
Ingredients:
- 2 garlic cloves, minced
- 1 teaspoon dried oregano, crushed
- 1 teaspoon dried basil, crushed

- Salt and ground black pepper, as required
- ¼ cup olive oil
- 2 tablespoons fresh lemon juice
- 4 (4-ounce) salmon fillets

Directions:
1. In a large bowl, add all ingredients except for salmon and mix well.
2. Add the salmon and coat with marinade generously.
3. Cover and refrigerate to marinate for at least 1 hour.
4. Place the water tray in the bottom of Power XL Smokeless Electric Grill.
5. Place about 2 cups of lukewarm water into the water tray.
6. Place the drip pan over water tray and then arrange the heating element.
7. Now, place the grilling pan over heating element.
8. Plugin the Power XL Smokeless Electric Grill and press the 'Power' button to turn it on.
9. Then press 'Fan" button.
10. Set the temperature settings according to manufacturer's directions.
11. Cover the grill with lid and let it preheat.
12. After preheating, remove the lid and grease the grilling pan.
13. Place the salmon fillets over the grilling pan.
14. Cover with the lid and cook for about 4 minutes per side.
15. Serve hot.

Nutrition Info: (Per Serving):Calories 263 ;Total Fat 19.7 g ;Saturated Fat 2.9 g ;Cholesterol 50 mg ;Sodium 91 mg ;Total Carbs 0.9 g ;Fiber 0.2 g ;Sugar 0.2 g ;Protein 22.2 g

Barbecue Squid

Servings: 4
Cooking Time: 3 Minutes

Ingredients:
- 1 ½ pounds skinless squid tubes, sliced
- ⅓ cup red bell pepper, chopped
- 13 fresh red Thai chiles, stemmed
- 6 garlic cloves, minced
- 3 shallots, chopped
- 1 (1-inch) piece fresh ginger, chopped
- 6 tablespoons sugar
- 2 tablespoons soy sauce
- 1 ½ teaspoons black pepper
- ¼ teaspoon salt

Directions:
1. Blend bell pepper, red chilies, shallots, sugar, soy sauce, black pepper and salt in a blender.

2. Transfer this marinade to a Ziplock bag and ad squid tubes.
3. Seal the bag and refrigerate for 1 hour for marination.
4. Turn the "Selector" knob to the "Grill Panini" side.
5. Preheat the bottom grill of Cuisine Griddler at 350 degrees F and the upper grill plate on medium heat.
6. Once it is preheated, open the lid and place the squid chunks in the Griddler.
7. Close the griddler's lid and grill the squid for 2-3 minutes.
8. Serve warm.

Nutrition Info: (Per Serving): Calories 248 ;Total Fat 15.7 g ;Saturated Fat 2.7 g ;Cholesterol 75 mg ;Sodium 94 mg ;Total Carbs 31.4 g ;Fiber 0.4 g ;Sugar 3.1 g ;Protein 24.9 g

Salmon Lime Burgers

Servings: 2
Cooking Time: 6 Minutes
Ingredients:
- 1-lb. skinless salmon fillets, minced
- 2 tablespoons grated lime zest
- 1 tablespoon Dijon mustard
- 3 tablespoons shallot, chopped
- 2 tablespoons fresh cilantro, minced
- 1 tablespoon soy sauce
- 1 tablespoon honey
- 3 garlic cloves, minced
- 1/2 teaspoon salt
- 1/4 teaspoon black pepper

Directions:
1. Thoroughly mix all the ingredients for burgers in a bowl.
2. Make four patties out this salmon mixture.
3. Turn the "Selector" knob to the "Grill Panini" side.
4. Preheat the bottom grill of Cuisine Griddler at 350 degrees F and the upper grill plate on medium heat.
5. Once it is preheated, open the lid and place the salmon burgers in the Griddler.
6. Close the griddler's lid and grill the salmon burgers for 6 minutes.
7. Serve warm with buns.

Nutrition Info: (Per Serving): Calories 408 ;Total Fat 21 g ;Saturated Fat 4.3 g ;Cholesterol 150 mg ;Sodium 146 mg ;Total Carbs 21.1 g ;Sugar 0.1 g ;Fiber 0.4 g ;Protein 23 g

Grilled Scallops

Servings: 4
Cooking Time: 6 Minutes
Ingredients:
- 1-pound Jumbo Scallops
- 1 ½ tbsp Olive Oil
- ½ tsp Garlic Powder
- Salt and Pepper, to taste
- Dressing:
- 1 tbsp chopped Parsley
- 3 tbsp Lemon Juice
- ½ tsp Lemon Zest
- 2 tbsp Olive Oil
- Salt and Pepper, to taste

Directions:
1. Preheat your grill to medium-high.
2. Brush the scallops with olive oi, and sprinkle with salt, pepper, and garlic powder.
3. Arrange onto the bottom plate and cook for about 3 minutes, with the lid off.
4. Flip over, and grill for an additional two or three minutes.
5. Meanwhile, make the dressing by combining all of the ingredients in a small bowl.
6. Transfer the grilled scallops to a serving plate and drizzle the dressing over.
7. Enjoy!

Nutrition Info: Calories 102 ;Total Fats 5g ;Carbs 3g ;Protein 9.5g ;Fiber: 1g

Grilled Garlic Scallops

Servings: 4
Cooking Time: 4 Minutes
Ingredients:
- 1/4 cup olive oil
- Juice of 1 lemon
- 3 garlic cloves minced
- 1 tablespoon Italian seasoning
- Salt and black pepper, to taste
- 1-pound scallops

Directions:
1. Mix Italian seasoning, black pepper, salt, garlic cloves, lemon juice and olive oil in a bowl.
2. Toss in scallops, mix gently, cover and refrigerate for 30 minutes.
3. Turn the "Selector" knob to the "Griddle" side.
4. Preheat the bottom grill of Cuisine Griddler at 350 degrees F.

5. Once it is preheated, open the lid and place the scallops in the Griddler.
6. Grill the scallop for 2 minutes flip and grill for 2 minutes.
7. Serve warm.

Nutrition Info: (Per Serving): Calories 351 ;Total Fat 4 g ;Saturated Fat 6.3 g ;Cholesterol 360 mg ;Sodium 236 mg ;Total Carbs 19.1 g ;Sugar 0.3 g ;Fiber 0.1 g ;Protein 36 g

The Easiest Pesto Shrimp

Servings: 2
Cooking Time: 5 Minutes
Ingredients:
- 1-pound Shrimp, tails and shells discarded
- ½ cup Pesto Sauce

Directions:
1. Place the cleaned shrimp in a bowl and add the pesto sauce to it.
2. Mix gently with your hands, until each shrimp is coated with the sauce. Let sit for about 15 minutes.
3. In the meantime, preheat your grill to 350 degrees F.
4. Open the grill and arrange the shrimp onto the bottom plate.
5. Cook with the lid off for about 2-3 minutes. Flip over and cook for an additional 2 minutes.
6. Serve as desired and enjoy!

Nutrition Info: Calories 470 ;Total Fats 28.5g ;Carbs 3g ;Protein 50g ;Fiber: 0g

Orange-glazed Salmon

Servings: 4
Cooking Time: 8 Minutes
Ingredients:
- 4 Salmon Fillets
- ½ tsp Garlic Powder
- 1 tsp Paprika
- ¼ tsp Cayenne Pepper
- 1 ¾ tsp Salt
- 1 tbsp Brown Sugar
- ¼ tsp Black Pepper
- Glaze:
- 1 tsp Salt
- 2 tbsp Soy Sauce
- Juice of 1 Orange
- 4 tbsp Maple Syrup

Directions:

1. Preheat your grill to medium and coat with cooking spray.
2. In a small bowl, combine the spices together, and then massage the mixture into the fish.
3. Arrange the salmon onto the bottom plate and cook with the lid off.
4. In the meantime, place the glaze ingredients in a saucepan over medium heat.
5. Cook for a couple of minutes, until thickened.
6. Once the salmon has been cooking for 3 minutes, flip it over.
7. Cook for another 3 minutes.
8. Then, brush with the glaze, lower the lid, and cook for an additional minute.
9. Serve with preferred side dish. Enjoy!

Nutrition Info: Calories 250 ;Total Fats 19g ;Carbs 7g ;Protein 22g ;Fiber: 0g

Lemon Pepper Salmon With Cherry Tomatoes And Asparagus

Servings: 4
Cooking Time: 5 Minutes
Ingredients:
- 4 Salmon Fillets
- 8 Cherry Tomatoes
- 12 Asparagus Spears
- 2 tbsp Olive Oil
- ½ tsp Garlic Powder
- 1 tsp Lemon Pepper
- ½ tsp Onion Powder
- Salt, to taste

Directions:
1. Preheat your grill to 375 degrees F and cut the tomatoes in half.
2. Brush the salmon, tomatoes, and sparagus with olive oil, and then sprinkle with the spices.
3. Arrange the salmon fillets, cherry tomatoes, and asparagus spears, onto the bottom plate.
4. Gently, lower the lid, and cook the fish and veggies for about 5-6 minutes, or until you reach your desired doneness (check at the 5th minute).
5. Serve and enjoy!

Nutrition Info: Calories 240 ;Total Fats 14g ;Carbs 3.5g ;Protein 24g ;Fiber: 1.4g

Simple Mahi-mahi

Servings: 4
Cooking Time: 10 Minutes
Ingredients:
- 4 (6-ounce) mahi-mahi fillets
- 2 tablespoons olive oil
- Salt and ground black pepper, as required

Directions:
1. Coat fish fillets with olive oil and season with salt and black pepper evenly.
2. Place the water tray in the bottom of Power XL Smokeless Electric Grill.
3. Place about 2 cups of lukewarm water into the water tray.
4. Place the drip pan over water tray and then arrange the heating element.
5. Now, place the grilling pan over heating element.
6. Plugin the Power XL Smokeless Electric Grill and press the 'Power' button to turn it on.
7. Then press 'Fan" button.
8. Set the temperature settings according to manufacturer's directions.
9. Cover the grill with lid and let it preheat.
10. After preheating, remove the lid and grease the grilling pan.
11. Place the fish fillets over the grilling pan.
12. Cover with the lid and cook for about 5 minutes per side.
13. Serve hot.

Nutrition Info: (Per Serving):Calories 195 ;Total Fat 7 g ;Saturated Fat 1 g ;Cholesterol 60 mg ;Sodium 182 mg ;Total Carbs 0 g ;Fiber 0 g ;Sugar 0 g ;Protein 31.6 g

Shrimp Skewers

Servings: 4
Cooking Time: 4 Minutes
Ingredients:
- 1/3 cup lemon juice
- 2 tablespoons olive oil
- 2 garlic cloves, minced
- 1/2 teaspoon lemon zest, grated
- 1 lb. uncooked shrimp, peeled and deveined
- Salt and black pepper, to taste

Directions:
1. Season the shrimp with olive oil, salt, black pepper lemon juice, lemon zest, oil, and garlic in a suitable bowl.
2. Thread the seasoned shrimp on the skewers.
3. And season the skewers with salt and black pepper.
4. Turn the "Selector" knob to the "Grill Panini" side.
5. Preheat the bottom grill of Cuisine Griddler at 350 degrees F and the upper grill plate on medium heat.
6. Once it is preheated, open the lid and place the shrimp skewers in the Griddler.
7. Close the griddler's lid and grill the skewers for 4 minutes.
8. Serve warm.

Nutrition Info: (Per Serving): Calories 338 ;Total Fat 3.8 g ;Saturated Fat 0.7 g ;Cholesterol 22 mg ;Sodium 620 mg ;Total Carbs 28.3 g ;Fiber 2.4 g ;Sugar 1.2 g ;Protein 15.4 g

Shrimp Kabobs

Servings: 6
Cooking Time: 8 Minutes

Ingredients:
- 1 jalapeño pepper, chopped
- 1 large garlic clove, chopped
- 1 (1-inch) fresh ginger, mined
- 1/3 cup fresh mint leaves
- 1 cup coconut milk
- ¼ cup fresh lime juice
- 1 tablespoon red boat fish sauce
- 24 medium shrimp, peeled and deveined
- 1 avocado, peeled, pitted and cubed
- 3 cups seedless watermelon, cubed

Directions:
1. In a food processor, add jalapeño, garlic, ginger, mint, coconut milk, lime juice and fish sauce and pulse until smooth.
2. Add shrimp and coat with marinade generously.
3. Cover and refrigerate to marinate for at least 1-2 hours.
4. Remove shrimp from marinade and thread onto pre-soaked wooden skewers with avocado and watermelon.
5. Place the water tray in the bottom of Power XL Smokeless Electric Grill.
6. Place about 2 cups of lukewarm water into the water tray.
7. Place the drip pan over water tray and then arrange the heating element.
8. Now, place the grilling pan over heating element.
9. Plugin the Power XL Smokeless Electric Grill and press the 'Power' button to turn it on.
10. Then press 'Fan" button.
11. Set the temperature settings according to manufacturer's directions.
12. Cover the grill with lid and let it preheat.
13. After preheating, remove the lid and grease the grilling pan.
14. Place the skewers over the grilling pan.
15. Cover with the lid and cook for about 3-4 minutes per side.
16. Serve hot.

Nutrition Info: (Per Serving):Calories 294 ;Total Fat 17.7 g ;Saturated Fat 10.4 g ;Cholesterol 185mg ;Sodium 473 mg ;Total Carbs 12.9 g ;Fiber 3.8 g ;Sugar 6.2 g ;Protein 22.9 g;

BEEF, PORK & LAMB RECIPES
Spiced Lamb Chops

Servings: 8
Cooking Time: 8 Minutes

Ingredients:
- 1 tablespoon fresh mint leaves, chopped
- 1 teaspoon garlic paste
- 1 teaspoon ground allspice
- ½ teaspoon ground nutmeg
- ½ teaspoon ground green cardamom
- ¼ teaspoon hot paprika
- Salt and ground black pepper, as required
- 4 tablespoons olive oil
- 2 tablespoons fresh lemon juice
- 2 racks of lamb, trimmed and separated into 16 chops

Directions:
1. In a large bowl, add all the ingredients except for chops and mix until well combined.
2. Add the chops and coat with the mixture generously.
3. Refrigerate to marinate for about 5-6 hours.
4. Place the water tray in the bottom of Power XL Smokeless Electric Grill.
5. Place about 2 cups of lukewarm water into the water tray.
6. Place the drip pan over water tray and then arrange the heating element.
7. Now, place the grilling pan over heating element.
8. Plugin the Power XL Smokeless Electric Grill and press the 'Power' button to turn it on.
9. Then press 'Fan" button.
10. Set the temperature settings according to manufacturer's directions.
11. Cover the grill with lid and let it preheat.
12. After preheating, remove the lid and grease the grilling pan.
13. Place the lamb chops over the grilling pan.
14. Cover with the lid and cook for about 6-8 minutes, flipping once halfway through.
15. Serve hot.

Nutrition Info: (Per Serving):Calories 380 ;Total Fat 19.6 g ;Saturated Fat 5.6 g ;Cholesterol 153 mg ;Sodium 150 mg ;Total Carbs 0.5 g ;Fiber 0.2 g ;Sugar 0.1 g ;Protein 47.9 g

Sweet Ham Kabobs

Servings: 6
Cooking Time: 7 Minutes
Ingredients:

- 1 can (20 oz.) pineapple chunks
- 1/2 cup orange marmalade
- 1 tablespoon mustard
- ¼ teaspoon ground cloves
- 1 lb. ham, diced
- ½ lb. Swiss cheese, diced
- 1 medium green pepper, cubed

Directions:
1. Take 2 tablespoons of pineapple from pineapples in a bowl.
2. Add mustard, marmalade, and cloves mix well and keep it aside.
3. Thread the pineapple, green pepper, cheese, and ham over the skewers alternatively.
4. Turn the "Selector" knob to the "Grill Panini" side.
5. Preheat the bottom grill of Cuisine Griddler at 350 degrees F and the upper grill plate on medium heat.
6. Once it is preheated, open the lid and place the skewers in the Griddler.
7. Close the griddler's lid and grill the skewers for 7 minutes.
8. Serve warm with marmalade sauce on top.
9. Enjoy.

Nutrition Info: (Per Serving): Calories 301 ;Total Fat 8.9 g ;Saturated Fat 4.5 g ;Cholesterol 57 mg ;Sodium 340 mg ;Total Carbs 24.7 g ;Fiber 1.2 g ;Sugar 1.3 g ;Protein 15.3 g

Fajita Skewers

Servings: 6
Cooking Time: 7 Minutes
Ingredients:
- 1 lb. sirloin steak, cubed
- 1 bunch scallions, cut into large pieces
- 1 pack flour tortillas, cut into triangles
- 4 large bell peppers, cubed
- olive oil, for drizzling
- Salt to taste
- Black pepper to taste

Directions:
1. Thread the steak, tortillas, peppers, and scallions on the skewers.
2. Drizzle salt, black pepper, and olive oil over the skewers.
3. Turn the "Selector" knob to the "Grill Panini" side.
4. Preheat the bottom grill of Cuisine Griddler at 350 degrees F and the upper grill plate on medium heat.
5. Once it is preheated, open the lid and place the fajita skewers in the Griddler.

6. Close the griddler's lid and grill the skewers for 7 minutes.
7. Serve warm.

Nutrition Info: (Per Serving): Calories 353 ;Total Fat 7.5 g ;Saturated Fat 1.1 g ;Cholesterol 20 mg ;Sodium 297 mg ;Total Carbs 10.4 g ;Fiber 0.2 g ;Sugar 0.1 g ;Protein 13.1 g

Rosemary Lamb Chops

Servings: 2
Cooking Time: 10 Minutes
Ingredients:
- 1 tablespoon olive oil
- 1 tablespoon fresh lemon juice
- 1 tablespoon fresh rosemary, chopped
- ½ teaspoon garlic, minced
- Salt and ground black pepper, as required
- 2 (8-ounce) (½-inch-thick) lamb shoulder blade chops

Directions:
1. In a bowl, place all ingredients and beat until well combined.
2. Place the chops and oat with the mixture well.
3. Seal the bag and shake vigorously to coat evenly.
4. Place the water tray in the bottom of Power XL Smokeless Electric Grill.
5. Place about 2 cups of lukewarm water into the water tray.
6. Place the drip pan over water tray and then arrange the heating element.
7. Now, place the grilling pan over heating element.
8. Plugin the Power XL Smokeless Electric Grill and press the 'Power' button to turn it on.
9. Then press 'Fan" button.
10. Set the temperature settings according to manufacturer's directions.
11. Cover the grill with lid and let it preheat.
12. After preheating, remove the lid and grease the grilling pan.
13. Place the lamb chops over the grilling pan.
14. Cover with the lid and cook for about 4-5 minutes per side.
15. Serve hot.

Nutrition Info: (Per Serving):Calories 410 ;Total Fat 25.4 g ;Saturated Fat 7.2 g ;Cholesterol 151 mg ;Sodium 241 mg ;Total Carbs 1.5 g ;Fiber 0.7 g ;Sugar 0.2 g ;Protein 44.3 g

Salisbury Steak

Servings: 5
Cooking Time: 12 Minutes
Ingredients:

- 1 1/2 pounds lean ground beef
- 1/2 cup seasoned breadcrumbs
- 1 tablespoon ketchup
- 2 teaspoons dry mustard
- 4 dashes Worcestershire sauce
- 1 cube beef bouillon, crumbled
- Salt and black pepper, to taste
- 1 tablespoon butter, melted

Directions:
1. Mix ground beef with breadcrumbs, ketchup, mustard, Worcestershire sauce, beef bouillon, butter, black pepper and salt in a bowl.
2. Make five patties out of the crumbly beef mixture.
3. Turn the "Selector" knob to the "Grill Panini" side.
4. Preheat the bottom grill of Cuisine Griddler at 350 degrees F and the upper grill plate on medium heat.
5. Once it is preheated, open the lid and place the patties in the Griddler.
6. Close the griddler's lid and grill the patties for 6 minutes.
7. Serve warm.

Nutrition Info: (Per Serving): Calories 548 ;Total Fat 22.9 g ;Saturated Fat 9 g ;Cholesterol 105 mg ;Sodium 350 mg ;Total Carbs 17.5 g ;Sugar 10.9 g ;Fiber 6.3 g ;Protein 40.1 g

Raspberry Pork Chops

Servings: 4
Cooking Time: 20 Minutes

Ingredients:
- 1/2 cup raspberry preserves
- 1 chipotle in adobo sauce, chopped
- 1/2 teaspoon salt
- 4 bone-in pork loin chops

Directions:
1. Take a small pan and mix preserves with chipotle pepper sauce on medium heat.
2. Keep ¼ cup of this sauce aside and rub the remaining over the pork.
3. Sprinkle salt over the pork and mix well.
4. Turn the "Selector" knob to the "Grill Panini" side.
5. Preheat the bottom grill of Cuisine Griddler at 350 degrees F and the upper grill plate on medium heat.
6. Once it is preheated, open the lid and place 2 pork chops in the Griddler.
7. Close the griddler's lid and grill the chops for 10 minutes.
8. Transfer them to a serving plate and grill remaining chops in the same manner.

9. Pour the reserved sauce over the pork chops.
10. Serve warm.

Nutrition Info: (Per Serving): Calories 401 ;Total Fat 50.5 g ;Saturated Fat 11.7 g ;Cholesterol 58 mg ;Sodium 463 mg ;Total Carbs 9.9 g ;Fiber 1.5 g ;Sugar 0.3 g ;Protein 29.3 g

Greek Souzoukaklia

Servings: 4
Cooking Time: 14 Minutes
Ingredients:
- 1 ½ pounds ground beef
- 1 onion, chopped
- ⅜ cup raisins, chopped
- 1 ½ teaspoons parsley, chopped
- ½ teaspoon cayenne pepper
- ½ teaspoon ground cinnamon
- ½ teaspoon ground coriander
- 1 pinch ground nutmeg
- ½ teaspoon white sugar
- Salt and black pepper to taste
- 1 tablespoon vegetable oil

Directions:
1. Mix ground beef with onion, raisins, and rest of the ingredients in a bowl.
2. Take a handful of this mixture and wrap it around each skewer to make a sausage.
3. Turn the "Selector" knob to the "Grill Panini" side.
4. Preheat the bottom grill of Cuisine Griddler at 350 degrees F and the upper grill plate on medium heat.
5. Once it is preheated, open the lid and place the skewers in the Griddler.
6. Close the griddler's lid and grill the skewers for 15 minutes.
7. Enjoy.

Nutrition Info: (Per Serving): Calories 361 ;Total Fat 16.3 g ;Saturated Fat 4.9 g ;Cholesterol 114 mg ;Sodium 515 mg ;Total Carbs 19.3 g ;Fiber 0.1 g ;Sugar 18.2 g ;Protein 33.3 g

Chimichurri Beef Skewers

Servings: 6
Cooking Time: 8 Minutes
Ingredients:
- 1/3 cup fresh basil
- 1/3 cup fresh cilantro

- 1/3 cup fresh parsley
- 1 tablespoon red wine vinegar
- Juice of 1/2 lemon
- 1 garlic clove, minced
- 1 shallot, minced
- 1/2 teaspoon crushed red pepper flakes
- 1/2 cup olive oil, divided
- Salt to taste
- Black pepper to taste
- 1 red onion, cubed
- 1 red pepper, cubed
- 1 orange pepper, cubed
- 1 yellow pepper, cubed
- 1 1/2 lb. sirloin steak, fat trimmed and diced

Directions:
1. First, take basil, parsley, vinegar, lemon juice, red pepper, shallots, garlic, and cilantro in a blender jug.
2. Blend well, then add ¼ cup olive oil, salt, and pepper and mix again.
3. Now thread the steak, bell peppers, and onion, alternately on the skewers.
4. Drizzle salt, black pepper, and remaining oil over the skewers.
5. Turn the "Selector" knob to the "Grill Panini" side.
6. Preheat the bottom grill of Cuisine Griddler at 350 degrees F and the upper grill plate on medium heat.
7. Once it is preheated, open the lid and place the skewers in the Griddler.
8. Close the griddler's lid and grill the skewers for 8 minutes.
9. Serve warm with green sauce.

Nutrition Info: (Per Serving): Calories 231 ;Total Fat 20.1 g ;Saturated Fat 2.4 g ;Cholesterol 110 mg ;Sodium 941 mg ;Total Carbs 20.1 g ;Fiber 0.9 g ;Sugar 1.4 g ;Protein 14.6 g

Spicy Pork Chops

Servings: 4
Cooking Time: 15 Minutes
Ingredients:
- 2 teaspoons Worcestershire sauce
- 1 teaspoon liquid smoke flavoring
- 1 tablespoon onion powder
- 1 tablespoon garlic powder
- 1 tablespoon paprika

- 1 tablespoon seasoned salt
- 1 teaspoon freshly ground black pepper
- 4 (½-¾-inch thick) bone-in pork chops

Directions:
1. In a bowl, mix together all ingredients except for chops.
2. Add chops and coat with mixture generously.
3. Set aside for about 10-15 minutes.
4. Place the water tray in the bottom of Power XL Smokeless Electric Grill.
5. Place about 2 cups of lukewarm water into the water tray.
6. Place the drip pan over water tray and then arrange the heating element.
7. Now, place the grilling pan over heating element.
8. Plugin the Power XL Smokeless Electric Grill and press the 'Power' button to turn it on.
9. Then press 'Fan" button.
10. Set the temperature settings according to manufacturer's directions.
11. Cover the grill with lid and let it preheat.
12. After preheating, remove the lid and grease the grilling pan.
13. Place the chops over the grilling pan.
14. Cover with the lid and cook for about 15 minutes, flipping once halfway through.
15. Serve hot.

Nutrition Info: (Per Serving):Calories 262 ;Total Fat 12.3 g ;Saturated Fat 4.1 g ;Cholesterol 85 mg ;Sodium 1800 mg ;Total Carbs 5.7 g ;Fiber 1.1 g ;Sugar 2.8 g ;Protein 29.9 g

Garlicky Flank Steak

Servings: 6
Cooking Time: 15 Minutes
Ingredients:
- 3 garlic cloves, minced
- 2 tablespoons fresh rosemary, chopped
- Salt and ground black pepper, as required
- 2 pounds flank steak, trimmed

Directions:
1. In a large bowl, add all the ingredients except the steak and mix until well combined.
2. Add the steak and coat with the mixture generously.
3. Set aside for about 10 minutes.
4. Place the water tray in the bottom of Power XL Smokeless Electric Grill.
5. Place about 2 cups of lukewarm water into the water tray.
6. Place the drip pan over water tray and then arrange the heating element.
7. Now, place the grilling pan over heating element.
8. Plugin the Power XL Smokeless Electric Grill and press the 'Power' button to turn it on.

9. Then press 'Fan" button.
10. Set the temperature settings according to manufacturer's directions.
11. Cover the grill with lid and let it preheat.
12. After preheating, remove the lid and grease the grilling pan.
13. Place the steak over the grilling pan.
14. Cover with the lid and cook for about 12-15 minutes, flipping after every 3-4 minutes.
15. Remove from the grill and place the steak onto a cutting board for about 5 minutes.
16. With a sharp knife, cut the steak into desired sized slices and serve.

Nutrition Info: (Per Serving):Calories 299 ;Total Fat 12.8 g ;Saturated Fat 5.3 g ;Cholesterol 83 mg ;Sodium 113 mg ;Total Carbs 1.2 g ;Fiber 0.5 g ;Sugar 0 g ;Protein 42.2 g

Prosciutto-wrapped Pork Chops

Servings: 4
Cooking Time: 14 Minutes
Ingredients:
- 4 (6-ounce) boneless pork chops
- Salt and ground black pepper, as required
- 8 fresh sage leaves
- 8 thin prosciutto slices
- 2 tablespoons olive oil

Directions:
1. Season the pork chops with salt and black pepper evenly.
2. Arrange 2 sage leaves over each pork chop.
3. Wrap each pork chop with 2 prosciutto slices.
4. Lightly brush both sides of chops with olive oil.
5. Place the water tray in the bottom of Power XL Smokeless Electric Grill.
6. Place about 2 cups of lukewarm water into the water tray.
7. Place the drip pan over water tray and then arrange the heating element.
8. Now, place the grilling pan over heating element.
9. Plugin the Power XL Smokeless Electric Grill and press the 'Power' button to turn it on.
10. Then press 'Fan" button.
11. Set the temperature settings according to manufacturer's directions.
12. Cover the grill with lid and let it preheat.
13. After preheating, remove the lid and grease the grilling pan.
14. Place the chops over the grilling pan.
15. Cover with the lid and cook for about 6-7 minutes per side.
16. Serves hot.

Nutrition Info: (Per Serving):Calories 384 ;Total Fat 16.1 g ;Saturated Fat 4.1 g ;Cholesterol 154 mg ;Sodium 809 mg ;Total Carbs 0.8 g ;Fiber 0 g ;Sugar 0 g ;Protein 56.2 g

Glazed Pork Chops

Servings: 6
Cooking Time: 12 Minutes

Ingredients:
- 2 tablespoons fresh ginger root, minced
- 1 teaspoon garlic, minced
- 2 tablespoons fresh orange zest, grated finely
- ½ cup fresh orange juice
- 1 teaspoon garlic chile paste
- 2 tablespoons soy sauce
- Salt, as required
- 6 (½-inch thick) pork loin chops

Directions:
1. In a large bowl, mix together all ingredients except for chops.
2. Add chops and coat with marinade generously.
3. Cover and refrigerate to marinate for about 2 hours, tossing occasionally.
4. Place the water tray in the bottom of Power XL Smokeless Electric Grill.
5. Place about 2 cups of lukewarm water into the water tray.
6. Place the drip pan over water tray and then arrange the heating element.
7. Now, place the grilling pan over heating element.
8. Plugin the Power XL Smokeless Electric Grill and press the 'Power' button to turn it on.
9. Then press 'Fan" button.
10. Set the temperature settings according to manufacturer's directions.
11. Cover the grill with lid and let it preheat.
12. After preheating, remove the lid and grease the grilling pan.
13. Place the chops over the grilling pan.
14. Cover with the lid and cook for about 10-12 minutes, flipping once in the middle way or until desired doneness.
15. Serve hot.

Nutrition Info: (Per Serving):Calories 560 ;Total Fat 42.3 g ;Saturated Fat 15.9 g ;Cholesterol 146 mg ;Sodium 447 mg ;Total Carbs 3.5 g ;Fiber 0.3 g ;Sugar 1.9 g ;Protein 38.8 g

Garlicky Marinated Steak

Servings: 1
Cooking Time: 8 Minutes

Ingredients:
- 4 Steaks (about 1 - 1 ½ pounds)

- 3 tbsp minced Garlic
- ¼ cup Soy Sauce
- 2 tbsp Honey
- ¼ cup Balsamic Vinegar
- 2 tbsp Worcesteshire Sauce
- ½ tsp Onion Powder
- Salt and Pepper, to taste

Directions:
1. Whisk together the garlic, sauces, and spices, in a bowl.
2. Add the steaks to it and make sure to coat them well.
3. Cover with plastic foil and refrigerate for about an hour.
4. Preheat your grill to high.
5. Open and add your steaks to the bottom plate.
6. Lower the lid and cook for about 4 minutes, or until the meat reaches the internal temperature that you prefer.
7. Serve as desired and let sit for a couple of minutes before enjoying!

Nutrition Info: Calories 435 ;Total Fats 24g ;Carbs 19g ;Protein 37g ;Fiber: 1g

Grilled Pork Chops

Servings: 4
Cooking Time: 20 Minutes
Ingredients:
- 4 pork chops bone in
- 1/4 cup olive oil
- 1 1/2 tablespoons brown sugar
- 2 teaspoons Dijon mustard
- 1 1/2 tablespoons soy sauce
- 1 teaspoon lemon zest
- 2 teaspoons parsley chopped
- 2 teaspoons thyme leaves, chopped
- 1/2 teaspoon salt
- 1/2 teaspoon black pepper
- 1 teaspoon garlic, minced

Directions:
1. Mix olive oil, brown sugar, Dijon mustard, soy sauce, lemon zest, parsley, thyme, salt, black pepper and garlic in a large and shallow bowl.
2. Add pork chops to the mixture and rub the spices all over.
3. Cover the pork chops and refrigerate for 1-8 hours for marination.
4. Turn the "Selector" knob to the "Grill Panini" side.

5. Preheat the bottom grill of Cuisine Griddler at 350 degrees F and the upper grill plate on medium heat.
6. Once it is preheated, open the lid and place 2 pork chops in the Griddler.
7. Close the griddler's lid and grill the pork chops for 10 minutes.
8. Cook the rest of the chops in the same way.
9. Serve warm.

Nutrition Info: (Per Serving): Calories 545 ;Total Fat 36.4 g ;Saturated Fat 10.1 g ;Cholesterol 200 mg ;Sodium 272 mg ;Total Carbs 40.7 g ;Fiber 0.2 g ;Sugar 0.1 g ;Protein 42.5 g

Filet Mignon

Servings: 2
Cooking Time: 10 Minutes
Ingredients:
- 2 filet mignons
- Salt and ground black pepper, as required

Directions:
1. Season the filet mignons with salt and black pepper generously.
2. Place the water tray in the bottom of Power XL Smokeless Electric Grill.
3. Place about 2 cups of lukewarm water into the water tray.
4. Place the drip pan over water tray and then arrange the heating element.
5. Now, place the grilling pan over heating element.
6. Plugin the Power XL Smokeless Electric Grill and press the 'Power' button to turn it on.
7. Then press 'Fan" button.
8. Set the temperature settings according to manufacturer's directions.
9. Cover the grill with lid and let it preheat.
10. After preheating, remove the lid and grease the grilling pan.
11. Place the filet mignons over the grilling pan.
12. Cover with the lid and cook for about 5 minutes per side.
13. Serve immediately.

Nutrition Info: (Per Serving):Calories 304 ;Total Fat 11.2 g ;Saturated Fat 4.3 g ;Cholesterol 112 mg ;Sodium 178 mg ;Total Carbs 0 g ;Fiber 0 g ;Sugar 0 g ;Protein 47.8 g

Maple Pork Chops

Servings: 1
Cooking Time: 7-8 Minutes
Ingredients:
- 4 boneless Pork Chops
- 6 tbsp Balsamic Vinegar

- 6 tbsp Maple Syrup
- ¼ tsp ground Sage
- Salt and Pepper, to taste

Directions:
1. Whisk the vinegar, maple, sage, and some salt and pepper in a bowl.
2. Add the pork chops and coat well.
3. Cover with plastic foil and refrigerate for one hour.
4. Preheat your grill to 350 degrees F.
5. Open and arrange the chops onto the bottom plate.
6. Lower the lid and cook closed for about 7 minutes, or until your desired doneness is reached.
7. Serve and enjoy!

Nutrition Info: Calories 509 ;Total Fats 19g ;Carbs 15g ;Protein 65g ;Fiber: 0g

Beef Skewers

Servings: 6
Cooking Time: 8 Minutes

Ingredients:
- 3 garlic cloves, minced
- 1 tablespoon fresh lemon zest, grated
- 2 teaspoons fresh rosemary, minced
- 2 teaspoons fresh parsley, minced
- 2 teaspoons fresh oregano, minced
- 2 teaspoons fresh thyme, minced
- 4 tablespoons olive oil
- 2 tablespoons fresh lemon juice
- Salt and ground black pepper, as required
- 2 pounds beef sirloin, cut into cubes

Directions:
1. In a bowl, add all the ingredients except the beef and mix well.
2. Add the beef and coat with the herb mixture generously.
3. Refrigerate to marinate for at least 20-30 minutes.
4. Remove the beef cubes from the marinade and thread onto metal skewers.
5. Place the water tray in the bottom of Power XL Smokeless Electric Grill.
6. Place about 2 cups of lukewarm water into the water tray.
7. Place the drip pan over water tray and then arrange the heating element.
8. Now, place the grilling pan over heating element.
9. Plugin the Power XL Smokeless Electric Grill and press the 'Power' button to turn it on.
10. Then press 'Fan" button.
11. Set the temperature settings according to manufacturer's directions.

12. Cover the grill with lid and let it preheat.
13. After preheating, remove the lid and grease the grilling pan.
14. Place the skewers over the grilling pan.
15. Cover with the lid and cook for about 6-8 minutes, flipping after every 2 minutes.
16. Remove from the grill and place onto a platter for about 5 minutes before serving.

Nutrition Info: (Per Serving):Calories 369 ;Total Fat 18.9 g ;Saturated Fat 5 g ;Cholesterol 135 mg ;Sodium 129 mg ;Total Carbs 1.6 g ;Fiber 0.6 g ;Sugar 0.2 g ;Protein 46.2 g

Spiced Pork Tenderloin

Servings: 6
Cooking Time: 18 Minutes
Ingredients:
- 2 teaspoons fennel seeds
- 2 teaspoons coriander seeds
- 2 teaspoons caraway seeds
- 1 teaspoon cumin seeds
- 1 bay leaf
- Salt and freshly ground black pepper, to taste
- 2 tablespoons fresh dill, chopped
- 2 (1-pound) pork tenderloins, trimmed

Directions:
1. For spice rub: in a spice grinder, add the seeds and bay leaf and grind until finely powdered.
2. Add the salt and black pepper and mix.
3. In a small bowl, reserve 2 tablespoons of spice rub.
4. In another small bowl, mix together the remaining spice rub, and dill.
5. Place 1 tenderloin onto a piece of plastic wrap.
6. With a sharp knife, slice through the meat to within ½-inch of the opposite side. Now, open the tenderloin like a book.
7. Cover with another plastic wrap and with a meat pounder, gently pound into ½-inch thickness.
8. Repeat with the remaining tenderloin.
9. Remove the plastic wrap and spread half of the spice and dill mixture over the center of each tenderloin.
10. Roll each tenderloin like a cylinder.
11. With a kitchen string, tightly tie each roll at several places.
12. Rub each roll with the reserved spice rub generously.
13. With 1 plastic wrap, wrap each roll and refrigerate for at least 4-6 hours.
14. Place the water tray in the bottom of Power XL Smokeless Electric Grill.
15. Place about 2 cups of lukewarm water into the water tray.

16. Place the drip pan over water tray and then arrange the heating element.
17. Now, place the grilling pan over heating element.
18. Plugin the Power XL Smokeless Electric Grill and press the 'Power' button to turn it on.
19. Then press 'Fan" button.
20. Set the temperature settings according to manufacturer's directions.
21. Cover the grill with lid and let it preheat.
22. After preheating, remove the lid and grease the grilling pan.
23. Remove the plastic wrap from tenderloins.
24. Place the tenderloins over the grilling pan.
25. Cover with the lid and cook for about 14-18 minutes, flipping occasionally.
26. Remove from the grill and place tenderloins onto a cutting board.
27. With a piece of foil, cover each tenderloin for at least 5-10 minutes before slicing.
28. With a sharp knife, cut the tenderloins into desired size slices and serve.

Nutrition Info: (Per Serving):Calories 313 ;Total Fat 12.6 g ;Saturated Fat 4.4 g ;Cholesterol 142 mg ;Sodium 127 mg ;Total Carbs 1.4 g ;Fiber 0.7 g ;Sugar 0 g ;Protein 45.7 g

Pork Burnt Ends

Servings: 1
Cooking Time: 6 Minutes

Ingredients:
- 1-pound Pork Shoulder
- 2 tbsp Favorite Rub Spice
- 2 tbsp Honey
- 1 ½ tbsp Barbecue Sauce

Directions:
1. Start by chopping the pork into cubes.
2. Place the meat in a bowl and add the spice, honey, and barbecue sauce.
3. With your hands, mix wel, making sure that each meat cube gets a little bit of honey, sauce, and spices.
4. Preheat your grill to 375 degrees F.
5. Arange the pork onto the bottom plate and lower the lid.
6. Cook for about 6 minutes.
7. Check the meat – if it is not too burnt for your taste, cook for an additional minute.
8. Serve as desired.
9. Enjoy!

Nutrition Info: Calories 399 ;Total Fats 27g ;Carbs 10.8g ;Protein 27g ;Fiber: 0g

Hawaian Kebobs

Servings: 4
Cooking Time: 6 Minutes

Ingredients:
- ½ cup Orange Juice
- 1 tbsp minced Garlic
- 1/3 cup Brown Sugar
- ½ tbs minced Ginger
- ½ cup Soy Sauce
- 1-pound Top Sirloin
- 1-pound Pineapple, fresh
- 2 Bell Peppers
- ½ Red Onion

Directions:
1. Place the first 5 ingredients in a medium bowl. Whisk to combine well.
2. Cut the steak into pieces and add to the bowl.
3. Stir well to coat, cover with plastic wrap, and place in the fridge for at least 60 minutes.
4. Meanwhile, cut the red onion, pineapple, and bell pepper, into chunks.
5. If using wooden skewers, soak them in cold water.
6. Preheat your grill to medium-high.
7. Thread the steak, pineapple, onion, and bell peppers onto the skewers.
8. Open the grill and arrange the skewers onto the bottom plate.
9. Cover, and let cook for 6 minutes.
10. Serve and enjoy!

Nutrition Info: Calories 460 ;Total Fats 13g ;Carbs 51g ;Protein 33g ;Fiber: 0.7g

Lamb Steak

Servings: 6
Cooking Time: 4 Minutes

Ingredients:
- 2 garlic cloves, minced
- 2 tablespoons olive oil
- 2 teaspoons dried oregano, crushed
- 2 tablespoons sumac
- 2 teaspoons sweet paprika
- 12 lamb cutlets, trimmed

Directions:
1. In a bowl mix together all ingredients except for lamb cutlets.

2. Add the cutlets and coat with garlic mixture evenly.
3. Set aside for at least 10 minutes.
4. Place the water tray in the bottom of Power XL Smokeless Electric Grill.
5. Place about 2 cups of lukewarm water into the water tray.
6. Place the drip pan over water tray and then arrange the heating element.
7. Now, place the grilling pan over heating element.
8. Plugin the Power XL Smokeless Electric Grill and press the 'Power' button to turn it on.
9. Then press 'Fan' button.
10. Set the temperature settings according to manufacturer's directions.
11. Cover the grill with lid and let it preheat.
12. After preheating, remove the lid and grease the grilling pan.
13. Place the cutlets over the grilling pan.
14. Cover with the lid and cook for about 2 minutes from both sides or until desired doneness.
15. Serve hot.

Nutrition Info: (Per Serving):Calories 343 ;Total Fat 16.6 g ;Saturated Fat 4.9 g ;Cholesterol 144 mg ;Sodium 122 mg ;Total Carbs 1 g ;Fiber 0.5 g ;Sugar 0.1 g ;Protein 45.2 g

Cheese Burgers

Servings: 4
Cooking Time: 8 Minutes

Ingredients:
- 1/2 cup cheddar cheese, shredded
- 6 tablespoons chili sauce
- 1 tablespoon chili powder
- 1-lb. ground beef

Directions:
1. First, take all the ingredients for patties in a bowl.
2. Thoroughly mix them together then make 4 of the ½ inch patties out of it.
3. Turn the "Selector" knob to the "Grill Panini" side.
4. Preheat the bottom grill of Cuisine Griddler at 350 degrees F and the upper grill plate on medium heat.
5. Once it is preheated, open the lid and place the patties in the Griddler.
6. Close the griddler's lid and grill the patties for 8 minutes.
7. Serve warm.

Nutrition Info: (Per Serving): Calories 537 ;Total Fat 19.8 g ;Saturated Fat 1.4 g ;Cholesterol 10 mg ;Sodium 719 mg ;Total Carbs 15.1 g ;Fiber 0.9 g ;Sugar 1.4 g ;Protein 37.8 g

Herbed Lemony Pork Skewers

Servings: 4
Cooking Time: 8 Minutes

Ingredients:
- 1-pound Pork Shoulder or Neck
- 1 tsp dried Basil
- 1 tsp dried Parsley
- 1 tsp dried Oregano
- 2 Garlic Cloves, minced
- 4 tbsp Lemon Juice
- ¼ tsp Onion Powder
- Salt and Pepper, to taste

Directions:
1. Start by soaking 8 skewers in cold water, to prevent the wood from burning on the grill.
2. Cut the pork into small chunks and place in a bowl.
3. Add lemon juice, garlic, spices and herbs to the bowl.
4. Give the mixture a good stir so that the meat is coated well.
5. Preheat your grill to medium-high.
6. Meanwhile, thread the meat onto the skewers.
7. When the green light turns on, arrange the skewers onto the bottom plate.
8. Cook for about 4 minutes per side (or more if you like the meat well-done and almost burnt).
9. Serve as desired and enjoy!

Nutrition Info: Calories 364 ;Total Fats 27g ;Carbs 1.6g ;Protein 26.7g ;Fiber: 0.1g

Grilled Lamb With Herbes De Provence

Servings: 6
Cooking Time: 18 Minutes

Ingredients:
- 1 rib (3 ounces-1-inch-thick) lamb chops
- 1/4 cups olive oil
- 2 lemons, juiced
- Salt and black pepper, to taste
- 3 tablespoons Herbes de Provence

Directions:
1. Rub the lamb chops with lemon juice, olive oil, black pepper, salt and Herbes de Provence.
2. Cover and marinate the chops for 1 hour in the refrigerator.
3. Turn the "Selector" knob to the "Grill Panini" side.

4. Preheat the bottom grill of Cuisine Griddler at 350 degrees F and the upper grill plate on medium heat.
5. Once it is preheated, open the lid and place half of the chops in the Griddler.
6. Close the griddler's lid and grill the chops for 9 minutes.
7. Transfer the grilled chops to a plate and grill the remaining chops in the same manner.
8. Serve warm.

Nutrition Info: (Per Serving): Calories 308 ;Total Fat 20.5 g ;Saturated Fat 3 g ;Cholesterol 42 mg ;Sodium 688 mg ;Total Carbs 40.3 g ;Sugar 1.4 g ;Fiber 4.3 g ;Protein 49 g

Pork Kabobs

Servings: 6
Cooking Time: 10 Minutes

Ingredients:
- 1 tablespoon smoked paprika
- 1 teaspoon onion powder
- ½ teaspoon garlic powder
- ¼ teaspoon cayenne pepper
- Salt and ground black pepper, as required
- 2 (¾-pound) pork tenderloins, trimmed and cut into 1-inch cubes
- ¼ cup balsamic vinegar
- 3 tablespoons honey
- 1 tablespoon Dijon mustard
- 2 teaspoons olive oil
- 12 dried figs, halved

Directions:
1. In a bowl, mix together the spices, salt and black pepper.
2. Add pork cubes and coat with the spice mixture generously.
3. Cover the bowl and refrigerate for about 30 minutes.
4. For glaze: in a bowl, place vinegar, honey, mustard and oil and beat until well combined.
5. Thread the pork cubes and fig halves onto pre-soaked wooden skewers.
6. Place the water tray in the bottom of Power XL Smokeless Electric Grill.
7. Place about 2 cups of lukewarm water into the water tray.
8. Place the drip pan over water tray and then arrange the heating element.
9. Now, place the grilling pan over heating element.
10. Plugin the Power XL Smokeless Electric Grill and press the 'Power' button to turn it on.
11. Then press 'Fan" button.
12. Set the temperature settings according to manufacturer's directions.
13. Cover the grill with lid and let it preheat.
14. After preheating, remove the lid and grease the grilling pan.

15. Place the skewers over the grilling pan.
16. Cover with the lid and cook for about 8-10 minutes, flipping and basting with glaze occasionally.
17. Serve hot.

Nutrition Info: (Per Serving):Calories 377 ;Total Fat 11.4 g ;Saturated Fat 3.6 g ;Cholesterol 107 mg ;Sodium 135 mg ;Total Carbs 34.3 g ;Fiber 4.3 g ;Sugar 27.2 g ;Protein 35.5 g

Steak Skewers With Potatoes And Mushrooms

Servings: 6
Cooking Time: 10 Minutes
Ingredients:
- 1-pound Steak
- 4 tbsp Olive Oil
- ½ pound Button Mushrooms
- 4 tbsp Balsamic Vinegar
- 1 pound Very Small Potatoes, boiled
- 2 tsp minced Garlic
- ½ tsp dired Sage
- Salt and Pepper, to taste

Directions:
1. Start by cutting the steak into 1-inch pieces.
2. Quarter the mushrooms.
3. Whisk the vinegar, oil, garlic, sage, and salt and pepper, in a bowl.
4. Add the meat, murshooms and potatoes to the bowl, coat well, and place in the fridge for 30 minutes. If your potatoes are not small enough for the skewers, you can chop them into smaller chunks.
5. In the meantime, soak the skewers in cold water.
6. Meanwhile, preheat your grill to medium-high.
7. Thread the chunks onto the skewers and arrange them on the bottom plate.
8. Keep the lid open and cook for 5.
9. Flip over and cook for 5 more minutes.
10. Serve and enjoy!

Nutrition Info: Calories 383 ;Total Fats 23g ;Carbs 21g ;Protein 23g ;Fiber: 3g

Grilled Lamb Chops

Servings: 6
Cooking Time: 18 Minutes
Ingredients:

- 2 large garlic cloves, crushed
- 1 tablespoon fresh rosemary leaves
- 1 teaspoon fresh thyme leaves
- Pinch cayenne pepper, to taste
- Sea salt, to taste
- 2 tablespoons olive oil
- 6 lamb chops, about 3/4-inch thick

Directions:
1. Rub the lamb chops with olive oil, garlic, rosemary, thyme, salt and cayenne pepper.
2. Cover the chops and marinate for 1-8 hours in the refrigerator.
3. Turn the "Selector" knob to the "Grill Panini" side.
4. Preheat the bottom grill of Cuisine Griddler at 350 degrees F and the upper grill plate on medium heat.
5. Once it is preheated, open the lid and place 3 chops in the Griddler.
6. Close the griddler's lid and grill the chops for 9 minutes.
7. Transfer them to a plate and grill the remaining chops in the same manner.
8. Serve warm.

Nutrition Info: (Per Serving): Calories 452 ;Total Fat 4 g ;Saturated Fat 2 g ;Cholesterol 65 mg ;Sodium 220 mg ;Total Carbs 23.1 g ;Fiber 0.3 g ;Sugar 1 g ;Protein 26g

Chipotle Bbq Ribs

Servings: 4
Cooking Time: 16 Minutes

Ingredients:
- 1-pound Back Ribs
- 3 tbsp Brown Sugar
- 1 ¾ cups BBQ Sauce
- 2/3 cups Balsamic Vinegar
- ½ tsp Chipotle Pepper
- ¼ tsp Garlic Powder
- Salt and Pepper, to taste

Directions:
1. Preheat your grill to 325 degrees F.
2. Sprinkle the ribs with salt, pepper, and garlic powder, and place on the bottom plate of the grill.
3. Cook for 8 minutes with the lid lowered.
4. In the meantime, combine the balsamic, BBQ sauce, sugar, and chipotle.
5. Lift the lid and sprinkle the mixture over the ribs.

6. Cook uncovered for about 8 more minutes, occasionally flipping over and adding more sauce as needed.
7. Serve and enjoy!

Nutrition Info: Calories 400 ;Total Fats 9g ;Carbs 75g ;Protein 7g ;Fiber: 1g

Margarita Beef Skewers

Servings: 6
Cooking Time: 10 Minutes
Ingredients:
- 1 cup margarita mix
- ½ teaspoon salt
- 1 tablespoon white sugar
- 2 garlic cloves, minced
- ¼ cup vegetable oil
- 1-pound top sirloin steak, cubed
- 16 mushrooms, stems trimmed
- 1 onion, cut into chunks
- 1 large red bell pepper, diced

Directions:
1. Mix margarita, salt, white sugar, garlic, vegetable, sirloin steak, mushrooms, onion, and red bell pepper on a bowl.
2. Cover and refrigerate the beef mixture for 1 hour for marination.
3. Thread the beef, mushrooms, onion and bell pepper, alternately on the wooden.
4. Turn the "Selector" knob to the "Grill Panini" side.
5. Preheat the bottom grill of Cuisine Griddler at 350 degrees F and the upper grill plate on medium heat.
6. Once it is preheated, open the lid and place the skewers in the Griddler.
7. Close the griddler's lid and grill the skewers for 10 minutes.
8. Serve warm.

Nutrition Info: (Per Serving): Calories 405 ;Total Fat 22.7 g ;Saturated Fat 6.1 g ;Cholesterol 4 mg ;Sodium 227 mg ;Total Carbs 26.1 g ;Fiber 1.4 g ;Sugar 0.9 g ;Protein 45.2 g

American Burger

Servings: 4
Cooking Time: 9 Minutes
Ingredients:
- 1/2 cup seasoned bread crumbs
- 1 large egg, lightly beaten

- 1/2 teaspoon salt
- 1/2 teaspoon pepper
- 1-lb. ground beef
- 1 tablespoon olive oil

Directions:
1. Take all the ingredients for a burger in a suitable bowl except the oil and the buns.
2. Mix them thoroughly together and make 4 of the ½ inch patties.
3. Brush these patties with olive oil.
4. Turn the "Selector" knob to the "Grill Panini" side.
5. Preheat the bottom grill of Cuisine Griddler at 350 degrees F and the upper grill plate on medium heat.
6. Once it is preheated, open the lid and place the patties in the Griddler.
7. Close the griddler's lid and grill the patties for 7-9 minutes.
8. Serve warm.

Nutrition Info: (Per Serving): Calories 301 ;Total Fat 15.8 g ;Saturated Fat 2.7 g ;Cholesterol 75 mg ;Sodium 389 mg ;Total Carbs 11.7 g ;Fiber 0.3g ;Sugar 0.1 g ;Protein 28.2 g

Flank Steak

Servings: 4
Cooking Time: 10 Minutes

Ingredients:
- 1/2 cup 1 tablespoon soy sauce
- 1/4 cup 2 tablespoon vegetable oil
- 1/2 cup rice wine vinegar
- 4 garlic cloves, minced
- 2 tablespoon ginger, minced
- 2 tablespoon honey
- 3 tablespoon sesame oil
- 3 tablespoon Sriracha
- 1 1/2 lb. flank steak
- 1 teaspoon sugar
- 1 teaspoon red pepper flakes
- 2 large cucumbers, sliced
- Salt to taste

Directions:
1. Mix ½ cup soy sauce, half of the rice wine, honey, ginger, garlic, 2 tablespoon Sriracha sauce, 2 tablespoon sesame oil, and vegetable oil in a large bowl.
2. Pour half of this sauce over the steak and rub it well.
3. Cover the steak and marinate for 10 minutes.

4. For salad mix cucumber with remaining rice wine vinegar, sesame oil, sugar, red pepper flakes, Sriracha sauce, soy sauce, and salt in a salad bowl.
5. Turn the "Selector" knob to the "Grill Panini" side.
6. Preheat the bottom grill of Cuisine Griddler at 350 degrees F and the upper grill plate on medium heat.
7. Once it is preheated, open the lid and place the steak in the Griddler.
8. Close the griddler's lid and grill the flank steaks for 10 minutes until done.
9. Serve warm with cucumber salad.

Nutrition Info: (Per Serving): Calories 327 ;Total Fat 3.5 g ;Saturated Fat 0.5 g ;Cholesterol 162 mg ;Sodium 142 mg ;Total Carbs 33.6 g ;Fiber 0.4 g ;Sugar 0.5 g ;Protein 24.5 g

Lamb Kabobs

Servings: 6
Cooking Time: 10 Minutes
Ingredients:
- 1 large pineapple, cubed into 1½-inch size, divided
- 1 (½-inch) piece fresh ginger, chopped
- 2 garlic cloves, chopped
- Salt, as required
- 16-24-ounce lamb shoulder steak, trimmed and cubed into 1½-inch size
- Fresh mint leaves from a bunch
- Ground cinnamon, as required

Directions:
1. In a food processor, add about 1½ cups of pineapple, ginger, garlic and salt and pulse until smooth.
2. Transfer the mixture into a large bowl.
3. Add the chops and coat with mixture generously.
4. Refrigerate to marinate for about 1-2 hours.
5. Remove from the refrigerator.
6. Thread lamb cubes, remaining pineapple and mint leaves onto pre-soaked wooden skewers.
7. Place the water tray in the bottom of Power XL Smokeless Electric Grill.
8. Place about 2 cups of lukewarm water into the water tray.
9. Place the drip pan over water tray and then arrange the heating element.
10. Now, place the grilling pan over heating element.
11. Plugin the Power XL Smokeless Electric Grill and press the 'Power' button to turn it on.
12. Then press 'Fan' button.
13. Set the temperature settings according to manufacturer's directions.
14. Cover the grill with lid and let it preheat.
15. After preheating, remove the lid and grease the grilling pan.
16. Place the skewers over the grilling pan.

17. Cover with the lid and cook for about 10 minutes, turning occasionally.

Nutrition Info: (Per Serving):Calories 288 ;Total Fat 8.5 g ;Saturated Fat 3 g ;Cholesterol 102 mg ;Sodium 115 mg ;Total Carbs 20.2 g ;Fiber 2.1 g ;Sugar 14.9 g ;Protein 32.7 g

Honey Glazed Pork Chops

Servings: 4
Cooking Time: 20 Minutes
Ingredients:
- 1/4 cup honey
- 1/2 cup low-sodium soy sauce
- 2 garlic cloves, minced
- Red pepper flakes, to taste
- 4 boneless pork chops

Directions:
1. Mix honey, soy sauce, garlic and red pepper flakes in a bowl.
2. Brush this honey mixture over the pork chops, liberally then marinate for 30 minutes.
3. Turn the "Selector" knob to the "Grill Panini" side.
4. Preheat the bottom grill of Cuisine Griddler at 350 degrees F and the upper grill plate on medium heat.
5. Once it is preheated, open the lid and place 2 pork chops in the Griddler.
6. Close the griddler's lid and grill the chops for 10 minutes.
7. Transfer these chops to a plate and grill the remaining chops in the same manner.
8. Serve warm.

Nutrition Info: (Per Serving): Calories 695 ;Total Fat 17.5 g ;Saturated Fat 4.8 g ;Cholesterol 283 mg ;Sodium 355 mg ;Total Carbs 26.4 g ;Fiber 1.8 g ;Sugar 0.8 g ;Protein 47.4 g

Lamb Skewers

Servings: 6
Cooking Time: 10 Minutes
Ingredients:
- 1 (10 oz.) pack couscous
- 1 1/2 cup yogurt
- 1 tablespoon 1 teaspoon cumin
- 2 garlic cloves, minced
- Juice of 2 lemons
- Salt to taste
- Black pepper to taste
- 1 1/2 lb. leg of lamb, boneless, diced
- 2 tomatoes, diced

- 1/2 English cucumber, diced
- 1/2 small red onion, chopped
- 1/4 cup parsley, chopped
- 1/4 cup fresh mint, chopped
- 3 tablespoon olive oil

Directions:
1. First, cook the couscous as per the given instructions on the package then fluff with a fork.
2. Whisk yogurt with garlic, cumin, lemon juice, salt, and black pepper in a large bowl.
3. Add lamb and mix well to coat the meat.
4. Separately toss red onion with cucumber, tomatoes, parsley, mint, lemon juice, olive oil, salt, and couscous in salad bowl.
5. Thread the seasoned lamb on 8 skewers and drizzle salt and black pepper over them.
6. Turn the "Selector" knob to the "Grill Panini" side.
7. Preheat the bottom grill of Cuisine Griddler at 350 degrees F and the upper grill plate on medium heat.
8. Once it is preheated, open the lid and place the lamb skewers in the Griddler.
9. Close the griddler's lid and grill the lamb skewers for 10 minutes.
10. Serve warm with prepared couscous.

Nutrition Info: (Per Serving): Calories 472 ;Total Fat 11.1 g ;Saturated Fat 5.8 g ;Cholesterol 610 mg ;Sodium 749 mg ;Total Carbs 19.9 g ;Fiber 0.2 g ;Sugar 0.2 g ;Protein 13.5 g

Teriyaki Beef Skewers

Servings: 6
Cooking Time: 6 Minutes

Ingredients:
- ¾ cup brown sugar
- ¼ cup soy sauce
- 1/8 cup pineapple juice
- 1/8 cup water
- 2 tablespoons vegetable oil
- 1 garlic clove, chopped
- 2 pounds boneless round steak, sliced

Directions:
1. Mix brown sugar, soy sauce, pineapple juice, water, vegetable oi, garlic cloves and steak slices in a bowl.
2. Cover and refrigerate the steaks for 24 hours for marination.
3. Thread the marinated beef on the wooden skewers.
4. Turn the "Selector" knob to the "Grill Panini" side.
5. Preheat the bottom grill of Cuisine Griddler at 350 degrees F and the upper grill plate on medium heat.
6. Once it is preheated, open the lid and place the skewers in the Griddler.

7. Close the griddler's lid and grill the skewers for 6 minutes.
8. Serve warm.

Nutrition Info: (Per Serving): Calories 380 ;Total Fat 20 g ;Saturated Fat 5 g ;Cholesterol 151 mg ;Sodium 686 mg ;Total Carbs 33 g ;Fiber 1 g ;Sugar 1.2 g ;Protein 21 g

Garlicy Lamb Chops

Servings: 4
Cooking Time: 6 Minutes
Ingredients:
- 1 tablespoon fresh ginger, grated
- 4 garlic cloves, chopped roughly
- 1 teaspoon ground cumin
- ½ teaspoon red chili powder
- Salt and ground black pepper, as required
- 1 tablespoon olive oil
- 1 tablespoon fresh lemon juice
- 8 lamb chops, trimmed

Directions:
1. In a bowl, mix together all ingredients except for chops.
2. With a hand blender, blend until a smooth mixture forms.
3. Add the chops and coat with mixture generously.
4. Refrigerate to marinate for overnight.
5. Place the water tray in the bottom of Power XL Smokeless Electric Grill.
6. Place about 2 cups of lukewarm water into the water tray.
7. Place the drip pan over water tray and then arrange the heating element.
8. Now, place the grilling pan over heating element.
9. Plugin the Power XL Smokeless Electric Grill and press the 'Power' button to turn it on.
10. Then press 'Fan" button.
11. Set the temperature settings according to manufacturer's directions.
12. Cover the grill with lid and let it preheat.
13. After preheating, remove the lid and grease the grilling pan.
14. Place the lamb chops over the grilling pan.
15. Cover with the lid and cook for about 3 minutes per side.
16. Serve hot.

Nutrition Info: (Per Serving):Calories 465 ;Total Fat 20.4 g ;Saturated Fat 6.5 g ;Cholesterol 204 mg ;Sodium 178 mg ;Total Carbs 2.4 g ;Fiber 0.4 g ;Sugar 0.2 g ;Protein 64.2 g

BREADS AND SANDWICHES
The Greatest Butter Burger Recipe

Servings: 6
Cooking Time: 11 Minutes
Ingredients:
- 2 pounds Ground Chuck Meat
- 1 ½ tsp minced Garlic
- 6 tbsp Butter
- 2 tbsp Worcestershire Sauce
- 1 tsp Salt
- ½ tsp Pepper
- 6 Hamburger Buns
- Veggie Toppings of Choice

Directions:
1. Preheat your grill to medium-high.
2. Meanwhile, place the meat, garlic, sauce, salt, and pepper, in a bowl.
3. Mix with your hands to incorporate well. Make six patties out of the mixture.
4. Into each patty, press about one tablespoon into the center.
5. Open the grill and coat with some cooking spray.
6. Arrange the patties onto the bottom plate and cook for 6 minutes.
7. Flip over and cook for 5 more minutes.
8. Serve in hamburger buns with desired veggie toppings.
9. Enjoy!

Nutrition Info: Calories 595 ;Total Fats 48g ;Carbs 25g ;Protein 27g ;Fiber: 1.5g

Simple Pork Chop Sandwich

Servings: 4
Cooking Time: 7 Minutes
Ingredients:
- 4 Hamburger Buns
- 4 Cheddar Slices
- 4 boneless Pork Chop
- Salt and Pepper, to taste
- 4 tbsp Mayonnaise

Directions:
1. Preheat your grill to 375 degrees F.
2. When the green light turns on, open the grill.
3. Season the pork chops with salt and pepper and arrange onto the bottom plate.

4. Lower the lid, and cook the meat closed, for about 5-6 minutes.
5. Open the lid and place a slice of cheddar on top of each chop.
6. Cook for another minute or so, uncovered, until the cheese starts to melt.
7. Spread a tbsp of mayonnaise onto the insides of each bun.
8. Place the cheesy pork chop inside and serve.
9. Enjoy!

Nutrition Info: Calories 510 ;Total Fats 30.6g ;Carbs 18.4g ;Protein 42g ;Fiber: 5g

Chicken Pesto Grilled Sandwich

Servings: 2
Cooking Time: 4 Minutes

Ingredients:
- 4 Slices of Bread
- 1 ½ cups shredded Mozzarella Cheese
- ½ cup Pesto Sauce
- 2 cups cooked and shredded Chicken Meat
- 8 Sundried Tomatoes
- 1 ½ tbsp Butter

Directions:
1. Preheat your grill to medium-high.
2. Combine the pesto and chicken in a bowl.
3. Brush the outsides of the bread with the butter.
4. Divide the pesto/chicken filling between two bread slices.
5. Top with sundried tomatoes and mozzarella cheese.
6. Open the grill and carefully transfer the loaded slices of bread onto the top bottom.
7. Top with the remaining bread slices, carefully.
8. Lower the lid, pressing gently.
9. Let the sandwiches cook for about 3-4 minutes, or until the desired doneness is reached.
10. Serve and enjoy!

Nutrition Info: Calories 725 ;Total Fats 44.5g ;Carbs 32g ;Protein 51g ;Fiber: 7.5g

Fish Tacos With Slaw And Mango Salsa

Servings: 4
Cooking Time: 6 Minutes

Ingredients:
- 4 Tortillas
- 1-pound Cod
- 3 tbsp butter, melted

- ½ tsp Paprika
- ¼ tsp Garlic Onion
- 1 tsp Thyme
- ½ tsp Onion Powder
- ½ tsp Cayenne Pepper
- 1 tsp Brown Sugar
- 1 cup prepared (or store-brought) Slaw
- Salt and Pepper, to taste
- Mango Salsa:
- ¼ cup diced Red Onions
- Juice of 1 Lime
- 1 Mango, diced
- 1 Jalapeno Pepper, deseeded and minced
- 1 tbsp chopped Parlsey or Cilantro

Directions:
1. Preheat your grill to medium.
2. Brush the butter over the cod and sprinkle with the spices.
3. When ready, open the grill, and arrange the cod fillets onto the bottom plate.
4. Lower the lid and cook for about 4-5 minutes in total.
5. Transfer to a plate and cut into chunks.
6. Place all of the mango salsa ingredients in a bowl and mix to combine.
7. Assemble the tacos by adding slaw, topping with grilled cod, and adding a tablespoon or so of the mango salsa.
8. Enjoy!

Nutrition Info: Calories 323 ;Total Fats 12g ;Carbs 31g ;Protein 24g ;Fiber: 3g

Buttery Pepperoni Grilled Cheese Sandwich

Servings: 2
Cooking Time: 5 Minutes
Ingredients:
- 4 slices of Bread
- 4 slices of Mozzarella Cheese
- 4 tbsp Butter
- 18 Pepperoni Slices

Directions:
1. Preheat your grill to medium-high.
2. Meanwhile, brush each slice of bread with a tablespoon of butter. It seems like too much, but the taste is just incredible.
3. Divide the mozzarella and pepperoni among the insides of two bread slices.

4. Top the sandwich with the other slices of bread, keeping the buttery side up.
5. When the green light appears, open the grill.
6. Place the sandwiches carefully onto the bottom plate.
7. Lower the lid, and gently press.
8. Allow the sandwich to cook for 4-5 minutes.
9. Open the lid, transfer to a serving plate, cut in half, and serve. Enjoy!

Nutrition Info: Calories 625 ;Total Fats 46g ;Carbs 29g ;Protein 22g ;Fiber: 2g

Cheesy Buffalo Avocado Sandwich

Servings: 4
Cooking Time: 4 Minutes
Ingredients:
- 1 Avocado
- 2 Bread Slices
- 2 slices Cheddar Cheese
- 1 tbsp Butter
- Buffalo Sauce:
- 4 tbsp Hot Sauce
- 1 tbs White Vinegar
- ¼ cup Butter
- ¼ tsp Salt
- 1 tsp Cayenne Pepper
- ¼ tsp Garlic Salt

Directions:
1. Preheat your grill to 375 degrees F.
2. Meanwhile, peel the avocado, scoop out the flash, and mash it with a fork.
3. Spread the avocado onto a bread slice, and top with the cheddar cheese.
4. Spread the butter onto the outside of the other bread slice.
5. Top the sandwich with the buttery slice, with the butter-side up.
6. Grease the bottom cooking plate and place the sandwich there, with the butter-side up.
7. Lower the lid, press, and let the sandwich grill for about 4 minutes.
8. Meanwhile, whisk together all of the sauce ingredients.
9. Serve the sandwich with the Buffalo sauce and enjoy!

Nutrition Info: Calories 485 ;Total Fats 24g ;Carbs 35g ;Protein 8g ;Fiber: 3g

VEGETARIAN RECIPES
Garlicky Mixed Veggies

Servings: 4
Cooking Time: 8 Minutes
Ingredients:
- 1 bunch fresh asparagus, trimmed
- 6 ounces fresh mushrooms, halved
- 6 Campari tomatoes, halved
- 1 red onion, cut into 1-inch chunks
- 3 garlic cloves, minced
- 2 tablespoons olive oil
- Salt and ground black pepper, as required

Directions:
1. In a large bowl, add all ingredients and toss to coat well.
2. Place the water tray in the bottom of Power XL Smokeless Electric Grill.
3. Place about 2 cups of lukewarm water into the water tray.
4. Place the drip pan over water tray and then arrange the heating element.
5. Now, place the grilling pan over heating element.
6. Plugin the Power XL Smokeless Electric Grill and press the 'Power' button to turn it on.
7. Then press 'Fan" button.
8. Set the temperature settings according to manufacturer's directions.
9. Cover the grill with lid and let it preheat.
10. After preheating, remove the lid and grease the grilling pan.
11. Place the vegetables over the grilling pan.
12. Cover with the lid and cook for about 8 minutes, flipping occasionally.

Nutrition Info: (Per Serving):Calories 137 ;Total Fat 7.7 g ;Saturated Fat 1.1 g ;Cholesterol 0 mg ;Sodium 54 mg ;Total Carbs 15.6 g ;Fiber 5.6 g ;Sugar 8.9 g ;Protein 5.8 g

Grilled Tofu With Pineapple

Servings: 4
Cooking Time: 8 Minutes
Ingredients:
- 1 pound firm Tofu
- 1 Red Bell Pepper
- 1 Yello Bell Pepper
- 1 Zucchini
- ½ Pineapple
- ½ tsp Ginger Paste
- Salt and Pepper, to taste
- 2 tbsp Olive Oil

Directions:
1. Preheat your grill to medium-high.
2. Meanwhile, chop the tofu and vegies into smaller chunks, and place in a bowl. If using wooden skewers, soak them into water before using.
3. Add ginger and oil to the bowl and mix until coated well.
4. Thread the veggies and tofu onto the skewers.
5. When the green light turns on, open the grill and arrange the skewers onto the bottom plate.
6. Cook for 4 minutes, then flip over and cook for additional four minutes.
7. Serve as desired and enjoy!

Nutrition Info: Calories 210 ;Total Fats 12g ;Carbs 9g ;Protein 12g ;Fiber: 2g

Vinegar Veggies

Servings: 4
Cooking Time: 10 Minutes
Ingredients:
- 3 golden beets, trimmed, peeled and sliced thinly
- 3 carrots, peeled and sliced lengthwise
- 1 cup zucchini, sliced
- 1 onion, sliced
- ½ cup yam, sliced thinly
- 2 tablespoon fresh rosemary
- 1 garlic clove, minced
- Salt and ground black pepper, as required
- 3 tablespoons vegetable oil
- 2 teaspoons balsamic vinegar

Directions:
1. Place all ingredients in a bowl and toss to coat well.
2. Refrigerate to marinate for at least 30 minutes.
3. Place the water tray in the bottom of Power XL Smokeless Electric Grill.
4. Place about 2 cups of lukewarm water into the water tray.
5. Place the drip pan over water tray and then arrange the heating element.
6. Now, place the grilling pan over heating element.
7. Plugin the Power XL Smokeless Electric Grill and press the 'Power' button to turn it on.
8. Then press 'Fan" button.
9. Set the temperature settings according to manufacturer's directions.
10. Cover the grill with lid and let it preheat.
11. After preheating, remove the lid and grease the grilling pan.
12. Place the vegetables over the grilling pan.
13. Cover with the lid and cook for about 5 minutes per side.
14. Serve hot.

Nutrition Info: (Per Serving):Calories 184 ;Total Fat 10.7 g ;Saturated Fat 2.2 g ;Cholesterol 0 mg ;Sodium 134 mg ;Total Carbs 21.5 g ;Fiber 4.9 g ;Sugar 10 g ;Protein 2.7 g

Basil Pizza

Servings: 2
Cooking Time: 7 Minutes
Ingredients:
- 1 pizza dough
- ½ tablespoon olive oil
- 1 cup pizza sauce
- 1½ cups part-skim mozzarella cheese, shredded
- 1½ cups part-skim provolone cheese, shredded
- 10 fresh basil leaves

Directions:
1. Place the water tray in the bottom of Power XL Smokeless Electric Grill.
2. Place about 2 cups of lukewarm water into the water tray.
3. Place the drip pan over water tray and then arrange the heating element.
4. Now, place the grilling pan over heating element.
5. Plugin the Power XL Smokeless Electric Grill and press the 'Power' button to turn it on.
6. Then press 'Fan" button.
7. Set the temperature settings according to manufacturer's directions.
8. Cover the grill with lid and let it preheat.
9. With your hands, stretch the dough into the size that will fit into the grilling pan.
10. After preheating, remove the lid and grease the grilling pan.
11. Place the dough over the grilling pan.
12. Cover with the lid and cook for about 2-3 minutes
13. Remove the lid and with a heat-safe spatula, flip the dough.
14. Cover with the lid and cook for about 2 minutes.
15. Remove the lid and flip the crust.
16. Immediately, spread the pizza sauce over the crust and sprinkle with both kinds of cheese.
17. Cover with the lid and cook for about 1 minute.
18. Remove the lid and cook for about 1 minute or until the cheese is melted.
19. Remove from the grill and immediately top the pizza with basil leaves.
20. Cut into desired sized wedges and serve.

Nutrition Info: (Per Serving):Calories 707 ;Total Fat 47.5 g ;Saturated Fat 23.1 g ;Cholesterol 80 mg ;Sodium 1000 mg ;Total Carbs 34.9 g ;Fiber 3.5 g ;Sugar 4.6 g ;Protein 35.8 g

Guacamole

Servings: 4
Cooking Time: 4 Minutes

Ingredients:
- 2 ripe avocados, halved and pitted
- 2 teaspoons vegetable oil
- 3 tablespoons fresh lime juice
- 1 garlic clove, crushed
- ¼ teaspoon ground chipotle chile
- Salt, as required
- ¼ cup red onion, chopped finely
- ¼ cup fresh cilantro, chopped finely

Directions:
1. Brush the cut sides of each avocado half with oil.
2. Place the water tray in the bottom of Power XL Smokeless Electric Grill.
3. Place about 2 cups of lukewarm water into the water tray.
4. Place the drip pan over water tray and then arrange the heating element.
5. Now, place the grilling pan over heating element.
6. Plugin the Power XL Smokeless Electric Grill and press the 'Power' button to turn it on.
7. Then press 'Fan" button.
8. Set the temperature settings according to manufacturer's directions.
9. Cover the grill with lid and let it preheat.
10. After preheating, remove the lid and grease the grilling pan.
11. Place the avocado halves over the grilling pan, cut side down.
12. Cook, uncovered for about 2-4 minutes.
13. Transfer the avocados onto cutting board and let them cool slightly.
14. Remove the peel and transfer the flesh into a bowl.
15. Add the lime juice, garlic, chipotle and salt and with a fork, mash until almost smooth.
16. Stir in onion and cilantro and refrigerate, covered for about 1 hour before serving.

Nutrition Info: (Per Serving):Calories 230 ;Total Fat 21.9 g ;Saturated Fat 4.6g ;Cholesterol 0 mg ;Sodium 46 mg ;Total Carbs 9.7 g ;Fiber 6.9 g ;Sugar 0.8 g ;Protein 2.1 g

Grilled Cauliflower

Servings: 4
Cooking Time: 40 Minutes

Ingredients:
- 1 large head of cauliflower, leaves removed and stem trimmed
- Salt, as required
- 4 tablespoons unsalted butter
- ¼ cup hot sauce
- 1 tablespoon ketchup
- 1 tablespoon soy sauce
- ½ cup mayonnaise

- 2 tablespoons white miso
- 1 tablespoon fresh lemon juice
- ½ teaspoon ground black pepper
- 2 scallions, thinly sliced

Directions:
1. Sprinkle the cauliflower with salt evenly.
2. Arrange the cauliflower head in a large microwave-safe bowl.
3. With a plastic wrap, cover the bowl.
4. With a knife, pierce the plastic a few times to vent.
5. Microwave on high for about 5 minutes.
6. Remove from the microwave and set aside to cool slightly.
7. In a small saucepan, add butter, hot sauce, ketchup and soy sauce over medium heat and cook for about 2-3 minutes, stirring occasionally.
8. Brush the cauliflower head with warm sauce evenly.
9. Place the water tray in the bottom of Power XL Smokeless Electric Grill.
10. Place about 2 cups of lukewarm water into the water tray.
11. Place the drip pan over water tray and then arrange the heating element.
12. Now, place the grilling pan over heating element.
13. Plugin the Power XL Smokeless Electric Grill and press the 'Power' button to turn it on.
14. Then press 'Fan" button.
15. Set the temperature settings according to manufacturer's directions.
16. Cover the grill with lid and let it preheat.
17. After preheating, remove the lid and grease the grilling pan.
18. Place the cauliflower head over the grilling pan.
19. Cover with the lid and cook for about 10 minutes.
20. Turn the cauliflower over and brush with warm sauce.
21. Cover with the lid and cook for about 25 minutes, flipping and brushing with warm sauce after every 10 minutes.
22. Transfer cauliflower to a plate and let cool slightly.
23. In a bowl, place the mayonnaise, miso, lemon juice, and pepper and beat until smooth.
24. Spread the mayonnaise mixture onto a plate and arrange the cauliflower on top.
25. Garnish with scallions and serve.

Nutrition Info: (Per Serving):Calories 261 ;Total Fat 22 g ;Saturated Fat 8.9 g ;Cholesterol 38 mg ;Sodium 1300mg ;Total Carbs 15.1 g ;Fiber 2.5 g ;Sugar 5.4 g ;Protein 3.3 g

OTHER FAVORITE RECIPES
Mexican Scrambled Eggs

Servings: 4
Cooking Time: 5 Minutes
Ingredients:
- 2 tablespoons vegetable oil
- 1 tomato, roughly chopped
- 1 spring onion, chopped
- 1 green chili, chopped
- 4 large eggs, beaten
- ¼ teaspoon Maldon salt

Directions:
1. Beat eggs with vegetable oil, tomato, spring onion, green chili, and Maldon salt in a bowl.
2. Open the top lid of the Cuisine Griddler and set the flat plate sides up.
3. Turn the "Selector" knob to the "Grill Panini" side.
4. Preheat the bottom plate of Cuisine Griddler at 350 degrees F and the upper plate on medium heat.
5. Once it is preheated, pour the egg mixture on both plates.
6. Stir and cook the eggs for 5 minutes until set.
7. Serve warm.

Nutrition Info: (Per Serving): Calories 138 ;Total Fat 11.8g ;Saturated Fat 2.9g ;Cholesterol 186mg ;Sodium 101mg ;Total Carbs 1.8g ;Fiber 0.3g ;Sugars 1.1g ;Protein 6.5g

Lamb Burgers

Servings: 5
Cooking Time: 16 Minutes
Ingredients:
- 2 pounds ground lamb
- 9 ounces Halloumi cheese, grated
- 2 eggs
- 1 tablespoon fresh rosemary, chopped finely
- 1 tablespoon fresh parsley, chopped finely
- 2 teaspoons ground cumin
- Salt and ground black pepper, as required

Directions:
1. In a large bowl, add all the ingredients and mix until well combined.
2. Make 10 equal-sized patties from the mixture.
3. Place the water tray in the bottom of Power XL Smokeless Electric Grill.

4. Place about 2 cups of lukewarm water into the water tray.
5. Place the drip pan over water tray and then arrange the heating element.
6. Now, place the grilling pan over heating element.
7. Plugin the Power XL Smokeless Electric Grill and press the 'Power' button to turn it on.
8. Then press 'Fan" button.
9. Set the temperature settings according to manufacturer's directions.
10. Cover the grill with lid and let it preheat.
11. After preheating, remove the lid and grease the grilling pan.
12. Place the burgers over the grilling pan.
13. Cover with the lid and cook for about 15-8 minutes per side.
14. Serve hot

Nutrition Info: (Per Serving):Calories 554 ;Total Fat 30.6 g ;Saturated Fat 15.9 g ;Cholesterol 269 mg ;Sodium 459 mg ;Total Carbs 2.3 g ;Fiber 0.4 g ;Sugar 1.5 g ;Protein 64.4 g

Grilled Watermelon Salad With Cucumber And Cheese

Servings: 4
Cooking Time: 4 Minutes

Ingredients:
- 1 Small Watermelon (approximately yielding 4 cups when cubed)
- 1 tbsp chopped Basil
- 1 Cucumber, chopped
- 3 ounces Feta Cheese, crumbled or cubed
- Juice of 1 Lime
- 1 tbsp Olive Oil
- Salt and Pepper, to taste

Directions:
1. Preheat your grill to medium.
2. Peel and slice the watermelon (discard any seeds).
3. Open the grill and arrange the watermelon onto the bottom plate.
4. Lower the lid and cook for 4 minutes.
5. Transfer to a cutting board and slice into chunks.
6. Place into a bowl and add the rest of the ingredients.
7. Toss well to combine and coat.
8. Serve and enjoy!

Nutrition Info: Calories 122 ;Total Fats 5g ;Carbs 17g ;Protein 4g ;Fiber: 1g

Italian Panini

Servings: 6

Cooking Time: 5 Minutes

Ingredients:
- 1 loaf rustic Italian bread, sliced
- 4 teaspoons honey mustard
- 12 ounces provolone sliced
- 4 ounces Black Forest ham, thinly sliced
- 4 ounces roast turkey breast, thinly sliced
- 4 ounces Genoa salami, thinly sliced
- 3 tablespoons butter, softened

Directions:
1. Place half of the bread slices on the working surface and brush the top with butter.
2. Divide the honey mustard, provolone, ham, turkey, salami over the bread slices.
3. Set the remaining bread slices on top of the salami.
4. Cut the sandwiches into half diagonally and brush the top with butter.
5. Turn the "Selector" knob to the "Grill Panini" side.
6. Preheat the bottom grill of Cuisine Griddler at 350 degrees F and the upper grill on medium heat.
7. Once it is preheated, place the sandwiches in the grill.
8. Close the griddler's lid and grill the panini for 5 minutes.
9. Serve warm.

Nutrition Info: (Per Serving): Calories 424 ;Total Fat 30.2g ;Saturated Fat 16.5g ;Cholesterol 104mg ;Sodium 1449mg ;Total Carbs 8.8g ;Fiber 0.4g ;Sugars 1.2g ;Protein 28.5g

Grilled Zucchini And Feta Salad

Servings: 4

Cooking Time: 3 Minutes

Ingredients:
- 1 Large Zucchini
- 1 cup Baby Spinach
- ½ cup crumbled Feta Cheese
- 1 cup Cherry Tomatoes, cut in half
- 1 cup Corn
- 3 tbsp Olive Oil
- 1 tsp Lemon Juice
- Salt and Pepper, to taste

Directions:
1. Preheat your grill to 350 degrees F.
2. Peel the zucchini and slice lengthwise. Season with salt and pepper.
3. Open the grill and coat with cooking spray.

4. Arrange the zucchini on top of the bottom plate and lower the lid.
5. Cook for 2-3 minutes.
6. Meanwhile, combine the remaining ingredients in a large bowl.
7. Transfer the zucchini to cutting bord and chop into pieces.
8. Add to the bowl and toss well to combine.
9. Serve and enjoy!

Nutrition Info: Calories 192 ;Total Fats 14.6g ;Carbs 12.6g ;Protein 5g ;Fiber: 2.7g

Vegan Scrambled Eggs

Servings: 4
Cooking Time: 8 Minutes
Ingredients:
- 1 package medium tofu, crumbled
- ¼ cup nutritional yeast
- 2 teaspoons garlic powder
- ½ teaspoons turmeric
- 1 teaspoon black salt
- ½ teaspoons black pepper
- 1 cup chicken broth

Directions:
1. Blend yeast, garlic powder, turmeric, black pepper, salt, broth in a blender.
2. Pour this mixture into a bowl and stir in crumbled tofu, then mix well.
3. Turn the "Selector" knob to the "Grill Panini" side.
4. Open the top lid of the Cuisine Griddler and set the flat plate sides up.
5. Preheat the bottom plate of Cuisine Griddler at 350 degrees F and the upper plate on medium heat.
6. Once it is preheated, add the tofu mixture to both plates.
7. Stir and cook the tofu mixture for 8 minutes until set.
8. Serve warm.

Nutrition Info: (Per Serving): Calories 73 ;Total Fat 2.3g ;Saturated Fat 0.5g ;Cholesterol 0mg ;Sodium 783mg ;Total ;arbs 6.7g ;Fiber 3.1g ;Sugars 0.7g ;Protein 8.7g

Chocolate Panini

Servings: 4
Cooking Time: 5 Minutes
Ingredients:
- 4 challah bread slices
- 2 ounces semisweet chocolate, chopped

Directions:
1. Place the 2 bread slices on the working surface and top the bread with chocolate.
2. Set the remaining bread slices on top and press gently.
3. Cut the sandwiches into half diagonally.
4. Turn the "Selector" knob to the "Grill Panini" side.
5. Preheat the bottom grill of Cuisine Griddler at 350 degrees F and the upper grill on medium heat.
6. Once it is preheated, place the sandwiches in the grill.
7. Close the griddler's lid and grill the panini for 5 minutes.
8. Serve warm.

Nutrition Info: (Per Serving): Calories 281 ;Total Fat 10.9g ;Saturated Fat 5.4g ;Cholesterol 0mg ;Sodium 327mg ;Total Carbs 44.1g ;Fiber 3.8g ;Sugars 19.9g ;Protein 5.7g

Spinach Scrambled Eggs

Servings: 6
Cooking Time: 5 Minutes

Ingredients:
- 2 oz full-fat yogurt
- 1 tablespoon olive oil
- 1 cup spinach, chopped
- 6 large eggs
- ⅓ cup cheddar cheese, shredded

Directions:
1. Beat eggs with olive oil, spinach, cheddar cheese, and yogurt in a bowl.
2. Open the top lid of the Cuisine Griddler and set the flat plate sides up.
3. Turn the "Selector" knob to the "Grill Panini" side.
4. Preheat the bottom plate of Cuisine Griddler at 350 degrees F and the upper plate on medium heat.
5. Once it is preheated, pour the egg mixture on both plates.
6. Stir and cook the eggs for 5 minutes until set.
7. Serve warm.

Nutrition Info: (Per Serving): Calories 124 ;Total Fat 9.4g ;Saturated Fat 3.2g ;Cholesterol 193mg ;Sodium 118mg ;Total Carbs 1.7g ;Fiber 0.1g ;Sugars 1.2g ;Protein 8.3g

Sausage Scrambled Eggs

Servings: 3
Cooking Time: 5 Minutes
Ingredients:

- 3 eggs
- ¼ cup milk
- Black pepper, to taste
- 2 ounces bulk pork sausage
- 2 bacon slices, chopped
- ¼ cup cooked ham, diced

Directions:
1. Beat eggs with milk, black pepper, pork sausage, and bacon in a bowl.
2. Open the top lid of the Cuisine Griddler and set the flat plate sides up.
3. Turn the "Selector" knob to the "Grill Panini" side.
4. Preheat the bottom plate of Cuisine Griddler at 350 degrees F and the upper plate on medium heat.
5. Once it is preheated, pour the egg mixture on both plates.
6. Stir and cook the eggs for 5 minutes until set.
7. Serve warm.

Nutrition Info: (Per Serving): Calories 224 ;Total Fat 16.4g ;Saturated Fat 5.4g ;Cholesterol 202mg ;Sodium 652mg ;Total Carbs 2g ;Fiber 0.2g ;Sugars 1.3g ;Protein 16.4g

CPSIA information can be obtained
at www.ICGtesting.com
Printed in the USA
LVHW101343030221
678263LV00004B/206